PA

AUTISM SPECTRUM DISORDER

How to Stop Yelling and Love More Children with Autism and ADHD! Peaceful Parent Strategies to Help Children with Special Needs to Overcome Challenges and Thrive

By

Jasper Hayward

TABLE OF CONTENTS

COPYRIGHT

This book:

POSITIVE PARENTING FOR AUTISM SPECTRUM DISORDER

How to Stop Yelling and Love More Children with Autism and ADHD! Peaceful Parent Strategies to Help Children with Special Needs to Overcome Challenges and Thrive

Written By

Jasper Hayward

This document aims to provide precise and reliable details on this subject and the problem under discussion.

The product is marketed on the assumption that no officially approved bookkeeping or publishing house provides other available funds.

Where a legal or qualified guide is required, a person must have the right to participate in the field.

A statement of principle, which is a subcommittee of the American Bar Association, a committee of publishers, and is approved. A copy, reproduction, or distribution of parts of this text, in electronic or written form, is not permitted.

The recording of this document is strictly prohibited. Any retention of this text is only with the written permission of the publisher and all liberties authorized.

The information provided here is correct and reliable, as any lack of attention or other means resulting from the misuse or use of the procedures or instructions contained therein is the total and absolute obligation of the user addressed.

The author is not obliged, directly or indirectly, to assume civil liability for any restoration, damage, or loss resulting from the data collected here. The respective authors retain all copyrights not kept by the publisher.

The information contained herein is solely and universally available for information purposes. The data is presented without a warranty or promise of any kind.

The trademarks used are without approval, and the patent is issued without the trademark owner's permission or protection.

The logos and labels in this book are the property of the owners themselves and are not associated with this text.

INTRODUCTION

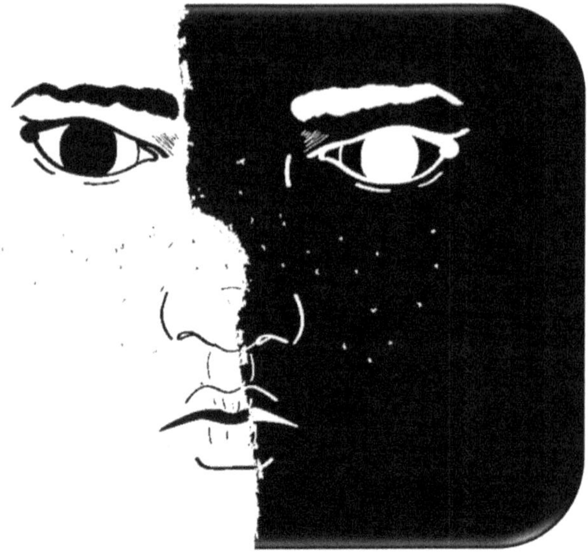

Being a parent doesn't mean how to discipline your kids effectively. It is mainly about nurturing their abilities, protecting them, understanding their feelings, and helping them deal with the world around them. We need to focus on helping and teaching them. The most effective way to learn is when your teacher is warm, thoughtful, and supportive; someone who gives you positive feedback on how well you are doing and corrects mistakes without being critical. For the first five years of life, your child is mainly learning from you.

You probably feel unsatisfied with how stressed you feel taking care of your preschooler. You are shouting more than you mean, you don't seem to like being with him due to constant requests; he never seems to listen to you and does not do as he is told. It's time to improve the quality of your relationship. First, you need to remember what you love about him rather than thinking about the problems. Make a list of all the things you like and like about your child. He can be very affectionate, have nice curly blonde hair, love looking at books, be cuddly, have a good sense of humor, have a good, contagious laugh. These are essential characteristics as they counteract all the problems you are facing, her hyperactivity, her tantrums, and her bedwetting. Despite his problems, you love him. Unfortunately, problems can begin to overshadow the positives, and it's easy to lose sight of the child you love.

You need to develop good qualities and improve your relationship with your child so that both of you enjoy being together. So, take time each day to be with him with no distractions or other work to do and no time pressures. The particular time is for you to rebuild your relationship, to help your child feel special and feel that his or her needs are recognized. If you're not used to praising your child, he needs practice. It may seem fake at first, but once you learn to notice the right things, it gets easier.

There can be a tremendous sense of joy and excitement in watching your child grow and develop. You quickly learn that your child is not a blank slate on which you write down your hopes and wishes for the future. He is an individual with his own needs to grow and learn, to investigate and explore. He wants to absorb the experiences of the world, and he needs you to modulate, protect, and help him cope with what happens. He is learning at a tremendous pace, but he thinks very differently from you. Many parents say, "It will be easier when he can talk, and I can reason with him," but in truth, if your child wants to do what he wants, no reasoning will stop him. So, please don't live in the false hope that it will get easier. He still won't listen to you. You are against willpower and an intoxicating sense of success and power when it gets its way.

CHAPTER NO 1: POSITIVE AND PEACEFUL PARENTS GROW JOYFUL CHILDREN

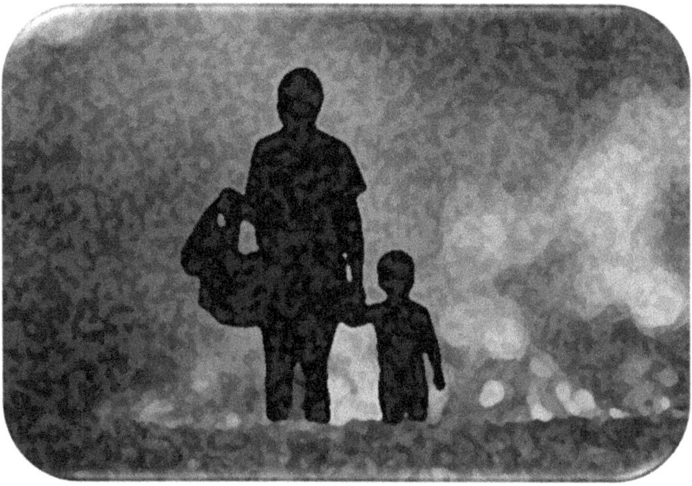

There is an old saying: raising children is the most challenging work there is. But why is it so difficult? Parents usually offer two reasons. First, the stakes are so high. And second, because there are no clear answers on how to do it right.

One answer is right, and the other is not. The stakes are undoubtedly high. But we know a lot about raising a happy, responsible, caring, emotionally healthy, and self-disciplined child. There is a great deal of valuable research on this most important topic, and parents will be happy to learn how reasonable it is. Time and again, studies show that parents who respond with a warm and respectful attunement to their individual child's unique needs. Also, sympathetically setting boundaries, and constructively educating their child's emotions, raising exceptional children. Sensitive but challenging. As any parent knows, the hard part is managing our emotional triggers to make it a reality sometimes too.

Regardless of your child's unique challenges, if you want to be a good parent, you need to work on yourself as well. A child does not cause the anger or anxiety that hooks us into power struggles, resulting from our fear and doubt. Our childhood experiences, our early, significant, and minor traumas, are part of who we are. Also, they are the part of us that takes charge whenever we are angry; so, when you are angry or scared, you know that it is almost always a bad early experience that drives your reactions. Babies have a way to unleash those unhappy feelings from our childhood, so the only way we can be peaceful parents is to prevent old feelings from causing new problems consciously.

The things we want most for our children depend on our inner work. We all want to raise children who are happy people, loved by others, and lucky in love. If we can reflect on our early childhood relationships and learn to nurture ourselves, we can offer our child, or you can offer your child a secure connection that will provide a foundation for loving relationships for the rest of their life. We can't control what happens to her. But we can get her to surround herself with people who treat her well and help her find profound meaning in her life.

We also want to raise children who know how to manage their behavior, both because it is easier to live with and our job as parents. We also know how to raise those children. When we regulate our emotions, our children learn to regulate their emotions. It allows them to regulate their behavior, assuming they are connected enough with us to want to.

Ultimately, we want our children to be successful, not necessarily in the sense of earning the rewards offered by our society for achievement, but in the sense of discovering, honing, and sharing their unique gifts for life. We also know how to help children do this. A lot has to do with managing our anxieties, which leaves our child-free to discover for themselves and build trust and resilience.

Some children are born with more difficult temperaments, and for those children, our inner work as parents is even more critical. Your baby will delight and exasperate you, excite you and annoy you. By chance, your child will ask you to grow up too. If you can notice when you are primed and restore balance before taking action, if you can soothe your anxiety, you can raise happy and emotionally healthy children who are successful in every sense. You can become a peaceful parent by raising happy children.

Responsibility as A Parent

Your child is sure that he is behaving like a child, which means that someone who is still learning has different priorities than yours and cannot always manage their feelings or actions. His childlike behavior is guaranteed, at times, to push your buttons. The problem is when we start acting like children too. Someone has to behave like an adult if we want our child to learn how! If, on the other hand, we manage to remain aware, that is, we notice our emotions and let them pass without acting on them, we model emotional regulation, and our children learn by observing us.

There's a reason airline tells us to put on our oxygen masks first. Children cannot reach for those masks or be reliable to use them properly. If we lose function, our children cannot save themselves or us. So even if we had to sacrifice ourselves to save our children, our responsibility is to put on our masks first.

Children cannot handle their anger alone. They can't find their way through the tangle of jealousy that drives them to beat up their little sister. They need our help dealing with the fear that we don't love them because, somehow, they aren't good enough. They know that if they were good enough, they wouldn't want to beat up their sister, or steal that piece of candy, or throw themselves down and scream. But they cannot help themselves, no matter how hard they try not to.

So, just like with the oxygen mask, it is your job to help your child with his emotions, which is what helps him with his behavior. Unfortunately, when you are stressed, exhausted, and running empty, you cannot be constructively there for your child any more than if you passed out on the plane.

That is why your first responsibility in parenting is to be aware of your inner state. Awareness is the opposite of "losing" patience. Don't get me wrong: awareness doesn't mean you don't feel anger. Being aware means paying attention to your feelings, but not acting accordingly. Anger is part of all relationships. Acting without thinking, with words or actions, is what compromises our parenting.

Emotions are useful, like the warning lights on a dashboard. If you saw a flashing red light in your car, you wouldn't cover it or tear the wiring that caused it, right? You would listen to the information and act on it, for example, taking your car for an oil change. The challenge with human emotions is that we are often confused about what to do when we feel them. We are programmed to respond to all "negative" emotions in one of three ways: fight, flight, or freeze.

These strategies work well in most emergencies. But parenting, despite our fears, is usually not an emergency. Usually, in parenting and life, the best response to upsetting emotions is to reflect, not react. In other words, don't take action while activated. You can count on finding yourself being hijacked by fight-or-flight hormones at times, but if you can train yourself to notice when you start losing it, you have a chance to return to a state of balance. That quiet place inside ensures that our actions are wise and loving.

But what happens when we can't get there? When something our child is doing is driving us crazy, and all our efforts to calm down don't work?

Wound Healing

Children don't need perfection from their parents. All we need to do is avoid harming them and offer them the "ordinary devotion" that has always been required of parents. Unfortunately, this isn't as easy as it sounds. First, there is nothing ordinary about devotion. Devotion, as parents know, is walking on the ground at 2:00 am holding a screaming child with an ear infection. Devotion is forcing yourself into the kitchen to make your child dinner after a long day when all you want is to curl up on the sofa and get out. Devotion takes off your jacket on a cold night to slip it around a sleeping child in the back seat of the car. This ordinary devotion is the same intense love that has led parents throughout human history to lash out between their child and danger, from flying glass to enemy soldiers.

The truth is that pretty much of us have been injured as children, and if we don't treat those injuries, they keep us from parenting our child the way we want. If there is an area where you were marked as a child, you can count on that area that causes you pain as a parent and injures your child in turn. We can all think of examples: the father unknowingly repeating his father's judgmental parenting with his son. The mother who cannot place limits on her children's behavior because she cannot bear their anger towards her, and ends up raising self-centered and anxious children. Parents who work too long hours because they doubt their care (translate: love) their children. For all of us, the task is to consciously examine our scars, some modest, some more painful, so as not to inflict new ones on our children.

The excellent news is that parenting gives us a map of where those scars are and a chance to dig deep and heal ourselves. Our children have an extraordinary ability to show us our wounded places, to bring out our fears and our anger. Better than the best Zen teacher or therapist, our children give us the perfect opportunity to grow and heal. Most parents say loving their children has transformed them: it has made them more patient, more compassionate, more selfless. We will always experience greater sensitivity around the problems that shaped our early psyche. Still, as we heal persistent wounds, our behavior is no longer guided by them, and we find that these scars inform us, motivate us, make us better parents. So how can you cure your childhood problems and become the parent you want for your children?

Parent Knowingly

If we pay attention, we will notice when our child presses our buttons. Not that kids don't act like kids, they always do. It is the appropriate age. But what bothers others would greet some parents with a calm, warm, and fun attitude that helps children want to behave. Whenever we are "triggered," we have stumbled upon something that needs healing. Seriously. Every time your child presses your buttons, it shows you an unsolved problem from your childhood.

Use Your Inner Button

You don't have to repeat the story with your children. Even if you are already on the wrong path, stop. Take a deep breath and press the pause button. Remind yourself what is going to happen if you don't choose another course. Shut your mouth, even in mid-sentence. Don't be embarrassed; you are modeling good anger management. Save yourself the embarrassment when you throw a tantrum.

Understand How Emotions Work

Anger is a message that something is wrong with our lives. The problem is that it is also a natural state that does not help us find the best solutions. When we are in the throes of chemical reactions that make us "angry," we do and say things we would never choose to do otherwise. When your body and emotions are in fight or flight mode, your child always looks like the enemy. Take a breath and wait to calm down before making any decisions or taking any action.

If you had a painful childhood, you can't change it. But what you can change is what you carry with you from that childhood: your "story." You do this by reflecting on it, experiencing the painful sensations, but also considering new angles. If your father left the family and you concluded that you weren't good enough, it's time to set the record straight and understand, from your adult point of view, that you were more than enough and that his departure had nothing to do. If your mother beat you and concluded that you were a bad boy, a more accurate understanding would be that your mother was scared and would hit even the most angelic child in the world. You were like any ordinary child: he sought love and attention in the only ways you knew. Coming to terms with your story and rewriting it can be a painful process, but it's liberating. It is also the only way to be the peaceful parent you want to be to your child. We all have a hard time being the parents we want to be when we're stressed out. Develop a repertoire of habits that help distract you: regular exercise, yoga, a hot bath, meditation. Can't find the time? Involve the whole family. Put on music and dance together, go for a walk, get everyone to bed with books early Friday nights for a quiet, relaxing evening, and catch up on sleep. Prioritize slowing down, and you'll find ways to do it.

Every parent needs support and an opportunity to talk about the hard work they are doing. Sometimes we can do this informally with friends or family. Sometimes a more formal "listening partnership" with another parent can be a lifesaver. You may want to be part of a parenting support group or community. If you feel stuck, find a counselor to help you move forward more happily in your life. There is no shame in asking for help; the shame would be to deny your responsibility as a parent by harming your child physically or psychologically. If you think you need help, don't wait. Get in touch now.

No parent is perfect because human beings are imperfect by definition. No matter how hard we work on ourselves, we won't always have a positive impact on our children. But every time you pay attention, press the inner pause button, and manage the stress, you become calmer. And this gives your child a greater chance of happiness. Our children don't need perfection from us. What they need is a parent who embraces growth, makes amends, and opens his heart when he wants to harden.

Managing the Anger

As long as you are human, you will sometimes find yourself in fight or flight mode, and your child will start to look like the enemy. When you are overwhelmed with anger, you are physically ready to fight. Hormones and neurotransmitters are flooding your body. They make the muscles contract, speed up the heartbeat, speed up the breath. It's impossible to stay calm in those spots, but we all know that beating up our kids while it can bring immediate relief isn't really what we want to do. So, commit now to not hitting, swearing, not calling your children, and not threatening. How about screaming? Never to your children; it's a whim. If you need to scream, get into the car with the windows closed and scream where no one can hear, and don't use words, because those make you angrier.

Your kids get angry too, so it's a double gift to them when you commit to constructive anger management. Not only do you not hurt them, but you offer them a model. Your children will surely see you angry from time to time, and the way you handle these situations will teach them a lot. Will you teach them it could do well? That even parents have tantrums? Is the anger part of being human and that learning to handle it responsibly is part of growing up? Here is how you can handle your anger:

Calm Yourself Down

Recognize that a state of anger is not the best place to intervene in any situation. Instead, give yourself a break and come back when you can be calm. If your child is old enough to be left for a moment, you can go to the bathroom, sprinkle water on your face, and breathe deeply. Just say, as calmly as possible, "I'm too angry right now to talk about it. I'll take a break and calm down. "Going out does not allow your child to win. It affects him how serious the infraction is and shapes self-control. If your child is small enough to feel abandoned when you leave, use the kitchen sink instead. So, sit on the sofa for a few minutes. Whether you are near your child or behind a closed door, use this time to calm down, so as not to get another frenzy about how right you are. A little mantra that restores calm. Your child will be watching. Don't worry about having to teach her a lesson about what she did wrong. She is receiving one of the most important lessons she will ever learn: regulating big emotions responsibly.

Help Your Body Release Anger

When you feel this angry, you need a way to calm down. Stop, breathe, remind yourself it's not an emergency. Shake the tension from your hands. Take ten deep breaths if you need to make noise, hum. You might try to find a way to laugh that releases tension and changes the mood. Forcing yourself to smile also sends a message to your nervous system that there is no emergency and start calming down. Touch the acupressure point on the side of one of your hands as you breathe and express your intention to calm down. If you feel you need to release your anger physically, put on some music and dance.

Time to Change Your Thoughts

If you think your child is spoiled who will grow up to be annoying, you can't calm down. The truth is that your child is a very young person who suffers, and he shows it to you with his behavior. Remind yourself: "He acts like a child because He is a child. My child needs my love most when he least" deserves "it. He asks for my help with his legitimate needs and feelings."

Understand Your Anger State and Act Accordingly

Anger, like other feelings, is as evident as our arms and legs. What we are responsible for is what we choose to do with it. Anger often has a valuable lesson for us. Still, to act while angry, except rare situations that require self-defense, it is rarely constructive, because we make choices that we would never make from a rational state. The constructive way to manage anger is to limit our expression of it and, when we calm down, use it diagnostically: what is so wrong with our life that it makes us angry and what do we need to do to change the situation? Sometimes the answer is related to our parenting, and we need to change our approach before things get out of hand, start putting the kids to bed half an hour earlier, or do some repair work on our relationship with our child. Nine years to stop treating us rudely. Sometimes we are surprised to find that our anger is towards our spouse, who does not act as a full partner in parenting, or even against our boss. Sometimes anger reminds us that we need to get more sleep or regularly let off steam with a friend who will accept the full range of our feelings. Sometimes, the answer is that we are carrying around anger that we do not understand pouring out on our children, and we need to seek help through therapy or a parent's support group.

Keep Your Anger to Yourself

Despite the popular idea that we must "express" our anger, so it doesn't devour us, research shows that expressing anger while angry makes us angrier. It makes the other person hurt, scared, or angry and causes a fracture in the relationship. Rethinking the situation in our mind always shows us that we are right and that the other person is wrong, which makes us even angrier as we get fed up. What works is to calm down and then find a constructive way to deal with whatever makes us angry so that the situation is resolved and our anger stops being triggered.

Constructive Disciplining

Nothing says you have to issue edicts on the fly. They will never be what's best for your child's long-term development, or even what's best to prevent a recurrence of the problem. Say as little as possible until you have calmed down, for example: "I need to calm down before I can talk about this." If you take a ten-minute break and still don't feel calm enough to relate constructively, you can say, "I want to think about what happened, and we'll talk about it later."

Avoiding Physical Force

Spanking can make you feel better temporarily because it dumps your anger, but it harms your child severely and ultimately sabotages the positive things you do as a parent. Spanking and even slapping have a way of escalating into harmful and sometimes even deadly violence. Do whatever it takes to control yourself, including leaving the room. If you can't control yourself and end up using physical strength, apologize to your child, tell him hitting is never okay, and get help.

Avoiding Threats

Threats made while you are angry will always be unreasonable. Since threats are only significant if you are willing to follow them, they undermine your authority and make it less likely that your child will follow the rules next time.

Choose Your Words

Research shows that the calmer we talk, the calmer we feel, and the calmer others respond to us. Similarly, the use of profanity or other positively charged words makes us and our listener more upset, and the situation escalates. We have the power to calm or upset ourselves and the person we are talking to with our tone of voice and choice of words.

You Are in It

If you are open to emotional growth, your child will always show you where you need to work on yourself. If you are not, you will find yourself trapped in the same vortex with your child over and over again. Your child may act in ways that irritate you, but you are not a helpless victim. Take responsibility for managing your emotions first. Your baby may not become an angel overnight, but his actions will drop once you learn to remain calm.

Don't Get Attached to Your Anger

After listening to it and making the appropriate changes, let it go. If that doesn't work, remember that anger is always a defense. It protects us from feeling vulnerable. To dissolve anger, look at the pain or fear underneath. If your daughter's whims scare you, or you are angry at your son for hitting his little sister because you were once the little sister who was beaten, reflect on those feelings and heal them. Once you are willing to experience the underlying feelings, you do not need the defense of anger, and it will dissolve.

Asking Advice

Each negative interaction with your child consumes a precious relationship capital. Focus on what matters, such as how your child treats other humans. In the larger scheme of things, his jacket on the floor might drive you crazy, but it’s probably not worth putting your bank account in the red.

CHAPTER NO 2: ELEMENTS OF PEACEFUL PARENTING

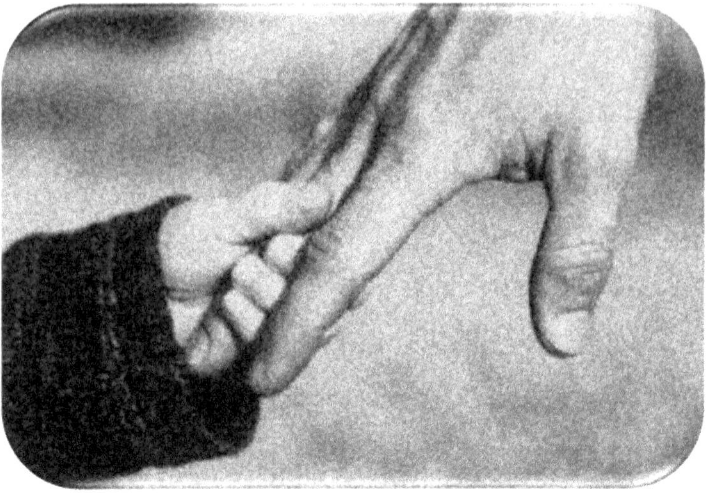

The security of knowing that someone is on his side, watching him, is what allows a child to risk bumps, scratches, and disappointment, in other words, to learn, grow and develop resilience. When children feel firmly connected to us, they learn to love themselves and to love others. The old saying that we give our children roots so they can later grow wings is more real than ever, and as always, it requires a secure bond for those roots to sink truly. Also, a good connection with your child is the key to being a happy parent. That's why Fostering Connection is one of the three big ideas at the heart of this book. As we shall see, our other two great ideas are also contained in the Fostering connection. Training, not controlling, is not possible if your children don't feel they are on their side in a profound and unspoken way. And when it comes to regulating yourself, your emotional integrity will determine how deeply you can connect with your child.

Connection

Sometimes parents approach connecting with their child as a duty. After all, we have a long list of obligations and what we want is an hour to ourselves without anyone throwing at us. But the truth is, that rewarding bond is our reward for all the hard work. The moments that make our hearts melt make all the right sacrifices worthwhile. And our children need to know that we feel joy in them or don't consider themselves worthy of being loved. Your ability to have fun with your child may be the most crucial factor in their development. It prompts you to automatically do all the things that help him thrive, from cooing in childhood to habitation at three and chatting at the age of five.

This deep connection is also what makes peaceful parenting possible. Children collaborate freely, even with enthusiasm, when they believe we are on their side. When they don't have this belief deep in their bones, our standards of behavior seem unfair, contradicting what they perceive as their best interest, whether it's taking the most significant piece of the pie or lying to us. No amount of "parenting skills" can compensate for an eroded parent-child bond. It's like riding a bike up a very steep hill.

Conversely, parenting with a good relationship is like going downhill. You still have to pay attention and stay on the road, and twists and turns undoubtedly arise, but the momentum is with you. A close bond gives us access to our natural parenting know-how and allows us to see things from our child's perspective, making us better parents. And it makes children more open to our influence, even as they move into the larger world of friends, school, and the rest of their lives. Study after study shows that the best protection for adolescents from cultural and peer group excesses is a close relationship with their parents. You have been building this connection since childhood.

Connect Deeply

Suppose you have to spend a significant amount of time building a good relationship with your child. Quality time is a myth because there is no switch to activate proximity. Imagine that you are working all the time and have reserved an evening with your husband, whom you have barely seen in the last six months. Does he immediately begin to bare his soul? It is not likely. In relationships, without quantity, there is no quality. You can't expect a good relationship with your daughter if you spend all your time at work and she spends all her time with friends, screens, or babysitter. As difficult as it is with the pressures of work and daily life, if we want a better relationship with our children, we need to free up time each day to make closeness possible.

We earn the trust of our children with our daily behavior. Keeping the promise, we make of playing a game with him, taking it on time, understanding even when he is not at his best. You don't have to do anything special to build a relationship with your child. The good and bad news is that every interaction creates a relationship. Shopping, carpooling, and a bath are at least as necessary as that big birthday party you planned for him. Doesn't she want to share her toy, or go to bed or do her homework? The way you face each challenge as he grows up is a building block of your relationship and his psyche. As much of our time with our children is about managing the activities of daily living, it's essential to make sure your routines are filled with fun, giggles, and warmth, rather than getting your child moving through the schedule. Play is one of the most reliable ways to relieve tension and build trust with your child.

Unfortunately, life, with its endless distractions and constant separations, has a way of eroding the connection. Work, school, technology, exhaustion, and the responsibility of keeping our children busy hours conspire to keep us from deeply connecting. The nursery is a separation, but so for a child, it's time to go to bed. In fact, for a young child, any time your attention is focused elsewhere is a separation. It is why they misbehave as soon as we call or start cooking dinner. Even when you take your child on errands, he may perceive your focus on the list and the store employees as a parting and acting out, demanding your attention.

That's why all parents have to repeatedly reconnect with their children, just to repair the daily erosion created by life's normal separations and distractions. Effective parenting is next to impossible until the positive connection with your child is re-established, so think of it as preventative maintenance before a problem arises. Parents naturally provide an anchor, or compass, for children to attach to and stay oriented. When they are away from us, they need a replacement, so they orient themselves around teachers, coaches, electronics, or colleagues. When you collect your child physically back into your orbit, you also collect them emotionally.

When to Work on The Relationship with Your Child

The most obvious sign that your relationship with your child needs some repair work is the challenge. Kids will always have different priorities than ours, but they want to feel good about their relationship with us, so they want to collaborate. When they don't, it's usually a sign of disconnection. So, the challenge is not a discipline problem. It's a relationship problem. Because young children are so forgiving and seek the approval and closeness of their parents at least sometimes, most parents say they have a good relationship with their children. We certainly know we love them, even if we lose patience. But by the time they're in their sixth grade, fewer than half of children in the United States describe their communication with their parents as positive. If you feel that you cannot communicate with your child; if your child does not listen or follow your requests or seems hardened by your anger; if you cry regularly, give "consequences" or pause your child, your relationship with your child's needs work. But even if your child seems complicated, he may be giving you the message that he needs something from you that he is not getting.

That doesn't mean you've somehow ruined your parenting. Many babies are harder to connect because they have colic, have a strong will, or were born with a specific challenge, such as a genetic predisposition to anxiety or depression. Other children encounter risk factors such as divorce, illness, separation, postpartum depression of a mother or sibling born while still children. The norm today for young children who spend a lot of time with non-parents simply doesn't work for all children. Many parents follow outdated parenting advice in their desire to do their best for their children. And our culture doesn't teach parents how to train emotions, so sometimes an emotional backpack overflowing with frustration or anxiety prevents a child from feeling close.

Finally, it is precisely like human relationships that we encounter conflicts with our child. In all these cases, a child can feel disconnected and act defiantly. It is always a sign that we need to do some repair work on the relationship.

It takes patience, the ability to regulate one's emotions, luck, and emotionally challenging work to mend a frayed relationship. The good news is, it's never too late to heal your bond with your child. Since separations and conflicts occur daily, small repairs must be a daily ritual. More extensive repairs require more concerted time and attention, and sometimes the help of a therapist, but they are always possible. No one can take your place in your child's heart; you will always be his parent. It may seem like she has hardened her heart with you, but your sweet little girl is there, waiting to be reunited with you.

Difficult Connection with Children

What if you have a child who doesn't seem to be motivated by connection? Children on the autism spectrum, or those with sensory processing problems such as ADHD, are good examples. These guys want to connect; you just have to be creative to find the ways to connect that work best. If your child fits this description, I urge you not to give up on the connection search. Pay close attention to how your child responds and adjust your attempts accordingly. What about the guys who are merely stimulating? Who looks like he's trying to chase you away by screaming and picking his nose and spitting on you? Believe it or not, those guys want to be close too. Indeed, the way to alleviate their problem behavior is actually to connect more, not less.

How to Stop Yelling at Your Child

Most parents scream. We don't even notice we do it half the time. Our voice gets louder and louder. Or we know we are doing it, but at that moment, it seems wholly justified. After all, did you see what that guy did? But we all know that our children respond better if we don't scream. Screaming intensifies a problematic situation, transforming it from a storm into a storm. And really, how can you expect your child to learn to control their emotions if you don't control yours?

If we manage to stay calm, everyone else calms down. We model emotional regulation. We can take action more effectively to solve the problem. Our baby learns to move on his own from troubled to calm. Our relationship with our son is strengthened. Collaborate more. Begin to control your emotions more.

And if we're honest, we know it's our things that make us scream. Some parents (really!) Would watch the same behavior and be able to remain empathetic or joke about it. Because no matter how bad your child's behavior is, it's a cry for help. Sometimes the behavior requires a firm boundary, but it never requires us to be wrong. And you can't help your child while you cry.

It's not easy to stop screaming. You may want it desperately and still find yourself screaming. If you've been yelled at, it takes tremendous work not to scream. But if you know you want to stop screaming, rest assured it's entirely possible no matter how ingrained it is. It is not rocket science. It takes about three months. How to learn to play the piano, you start playing the scales today, you practice daily, and soon you can choose simple pieces. In a year, you can play a sonata. I've seen hundreds of parents do it.

Will it be hard to stop screaming? Yes. It doesn't happen like magic. It takes a constant and daily effort. Nobody can do it for you. Not screaming may seem like a miracle, but it's something you can do. If you keep working on it, one day you will suddenly realize that you can't remember the last time you yelled. Here are the things you need to understand.

Commitment Making

When we verbally and consciously "commit" to a course of action, we are likely to realize it, primarily if we work on it daily. Conversely, simply "wanting" something would be different, or even "regretting" the things we have done, usually doesn't change anything. Then write your intention ("I will speak respectfully to my child") and post it in a place where you will see it often. Imagine how beautiful it will be in your home when you're not screaming. Imagine responding calmly, perhaps even empathically, or with a sense of humor! To the things, you scream about today. Keep revisiting that image. You are programming your subconscious.

There Is A Problem

Somehow you have to commit to someone else. Specifically, you need to commit your child to stop screaming because your child is the only person who will be there to keep you honest. A little scary? Yes. But you are a role model, and if you want a child who doesn't scold you, this is the way to get there. Then tell your kids that you have decided to stop screaming.

Stop, Breath, And Keep Patience

Stop, drop, and breathe every time you find yourself raising your voice or raising your voice. Stop talking as soon as you find yourself losing patience. Shut up. Can't stop making noise? Hum, if you have to. Breathe deeply ten times. Shake your hands. It moves you out of your "reptilian brain" - the fight, flight, or freeze response - and into conscious presence. Now you can choose how to act.

Forget It

Really! Forget it for now. It is not an emergency. If it is, get everyone out of harm's way and then go back to this process. Step away from the situation.

Do Whatever Calms You Down

You are an adult, and your child is learning from everything you do right now. Look at your son and say, "I'm working hard to keep calm. I don't want to scream. Let me calm down, and then we'll try to do it again, okay?" Do whatever works to calm your body's fight or flight response: breathe deeper, say a mantra, sprinkle cold water on your face, look at the sticker chart of your respectful voice, remind yourself that your child acts like a child because he is a child. Remind yourself that there is no emergency.

When you are out of the fight or flight, you will know this because your child will no longer look like the enemy, but like your beloved child, the one you promised to love, love, and lead so that he grows into a loving and wonderful person. Now, start the interaction again. Difficult, right? Very difficult when you are run over by neurochemicals that tell you to attack. But simple, you delay the interaction until you are calm.

- Wondering how your child will learn if you don't raise your voice? When children are afraid, they go into fight or flight. The learning centers of the brain shut down. Your child cannot learn when you scream. It is always more effective to intervene with calm and compassion. Also, when you scream, you lose credibility with your child. Children become less open to your influence.
- Wondering if maybe you are letting your child go too quickly? He is in pain, and his "misbehavior" is an SOS who needs your help. He is acting because he has excellent feelings that he cannot yet verbally understand and articulate. You set limits and redirect behavior.

But you're driving must never be wrong or scary. You want your child to follow your lead because he loves you and would never want to disappoint you, not because you scare him.

- Wondering if you are not authentic? Your son saw that you were very upset. He also saw that you were responsible for managing your emotions. Being authentic about the truth of your experience never requires you to "dump" them on someone else, unfiltered. It is always possible. "Also, it's your feelings, and only part of the emotion comes from this current interaction with your child. Most of it comes from your past and how you view this situation.
- What if you find yourself screaming despite your best efforts? You will do this in the beginning, more than once.

But it's not a mistake if you learn from it. Use whenever you miss the mark as an opportunity to change something about your routine, your attitude, or your self-care. So, you can do better next time. Support yourself so you can change.

Keep Yourself Calm

Children often get angry due to their inexperience and cognitive immaturity. We can remain calm when they are upset, helping them develop the neural pathways to calm down. But most of us find it challenging to remain empathetic when our child starts losing her. Something in us wants to shout "No!" and repeatedly, you say:

- No, I don't have time for this right now!
- No, you are embarrassing me; people are looking for!

- No, what am I doing wrong with her having tantrums again?
- No, why are you doing this to me?

Most of us learned as children that our feelings were unacceptable, even dangerous. So, when our child has a breakdown, the little one inside us is triggered. The warning signs flash. As always, when danger looms, we feel a sense of panic. We want to run away (flight), or we experience a wave of sudden anger, we want to silence him (fight), or we go numb (freezing). Holding him with empathy, allowing him to let out all those feelings? Accept his outburst even when it is directed at us, without taking it personally? It's a stretch for most parents. All our good intentions fly out the window.

Yet every child has numerous experiences of fear, anger, frustration, and sadness. They have to express those experiences and make us listen. Over time, this teaches them to befriend their emotions so they can handle them. Indeed, we are the role model. Our baby learns to regulate his emotions and behavior by observing us regulate our emotions and behavior. What can we do to address our profound reaction to our child's upset so that we can be there for our children?

Acknowledge Your Feelings

Our panic in the face of our child's raw emotions is a problem from our childhood. The only way to eradicate it is to see how it served us when we were little. Tell your growing panic: "Thank you for keeping me safe when I was little. I have grown up now. These feelings are okay. "

Remind Yourself That This Is Not an Emergency

"It's only natural that I feel this way when my son is angry. But whatever happens, I can handle it." It isn't a threat; it is your beloved child who needs your loving help right now. If your mind is so persistent in setting off alarms, tell her you will address these concerns later, not now.

Remind Yourself That Expressing Feelings Is A Good Thing

Your child will have these feelings, no matter what happens. The only question is whether you do well to express them or teach him that they are dangerous. Once he feels his emotions, they will fade away. (If you're wondering, it's the emotions he represses that pop up without warning and make him act out.) Even if you can't say a wholehearted, yes! When your child starts to melt, try moving away from your automatic no! to a loving okay, just like you do other times when your child needs you.

Release the Pressure

You don't have to fix your child or the situation. All you have to do is stay there. Your child doesn't even need the red cup, or whatever is crying; he needs your loving acceptance of him, complete with all his tangled feelings. His disappointment, anger, pain? They are all fine, and they will all go by without you doing anything except loving him.

Take A Deep Breath and Choose Love

Every choice we make, after all, is a movement towards love or fear. Let your care for your child give you the courage to choose love. Not just love for your child, but love for the child you once were and the parent you are now. Keep breathing and saying to yourself: "I choose love." Too trivial?

Tolerate Emotion Without Acting

You can act later if you want. Or even in a few minutes once you've calmed down. For now, let yourself be heard. Breathe through it. Name the emotion if that helps. Okay, anger. But what's underneath the anger? Bad? Fear? Disappointment? Notice how it feels in your body.

Be Simple

Your child needs you to witness her emotional outburst and let her know she is still adorable, despite all these awful feelings. Explanations, negotiations, remorse, recriminations, advice, analysis of why she is so upset or attempts to "comfort her (There, you don't have to cry, that's enough)." here, you don't have to cry, that's enough," will interrupt this natural emotional process. Do not force her to put into words; she has no access to the rational brain when she is so upset. Sure, you want to teach, but you have to wait. Your child cannot learn until she is calm. Your calm, loving tone is what matters.

Find A Way to Process Your Feelings

Nothing triggers primal emotions like parenting. You also have to let off steam, which means feeling those emotions and breathing through them without taking action. Some of us may do this by journaling or crying, but you may need to find someone who just listens to you. Someone who will resist giving you advice. Someone who won't be shocked when you admit that you wanted to bump your kid into the wall or leave him there in the grocery store because they know everyone has felt this way, and you really wouldn't. Someone who won't trigger and panic that it's okay for you, or your child, to try these things. Someone who will let you cry, who will be there for you just like you are there for your child.

It is hard work for parents, but an excellent gift for our children. The good news is that once we say yes to the full range of children's feelings, they learn to manage them healthily. You will see positive results immediately after every "whim" you meet with love because your child will feel so much better after emptying that backpack full of feelings. It is unconditional love in action.

Raise Yourself as You Raise Your Child

The number one resolution of parents everywhere? Be more patient. But having to call for patience is a sign that your cup is already dangerously empty. Willpower only takes us so far. The real job is keeping the cup full so that you have a lot of joy and presence to share with your child. Children love our joyful presence and become happier and more cooperative. If you often find yourself resentful, impoverished, or exhausted, if you often have negative thoughts about your child, or if you regularly yell at your child, you may be suffering from SAP disorder: sacrificing yourself on the altar of parenthood. That's when we forget to give ourselves the attention we need. It is not suitable for us to feel deprived. It kills our natural joy. And it's not suitable for our children, who end up having a resentful, cynical, and impatient parent.

Ultimately, you are in charge of how you spend the short life assigned to you. On your deathbed, there will be no one else to blame if you have been unhappy. The secret job of adulthood is that we are still growing up, and parenting forces us to learn to be parents ourselves and our child. If you are old enough to have a child on your own, your parents are off the hook. Now it is your responsibility. You deserve all the tenderness you would shower on a newborn. Giving that love to ourselves transforms our parenting and our life. Does this mean that you should tell your child that he can forget to get his needs met, that it is time for your needs to come first? No, of course not. Parenting means feeding your child, which means noticing what he needs and making sure he gets it. After all, you are an adult. But we can be peaceful parents only to the extent that we "assure" ourselves.

It's partly a matter of changing what you do: feeding yourself in small ways throughout the day. And it's partly a matter of changing your attitude: finding peace within yourself. The solution is to take care of ourselves in the best possible way at any time of the day, just like we do with our child. The bad news is that this takes work. But that work, the internal work of embracing us with compassion, is what transforms us. Here's how you do it:

Tune Yourself Throughout the Day

Take a deep breath and let it flood your body with well-being. Breathe calmly, exhale the stress. Simply being present with yourself is a necessary form of "attention" that we all need.

When You Are Resentful, Stop

Ask yourself, "What do I need now to stay balanced?" So, give it to yourself, whether your child is present or not. Five minutes to sit on the back steps and listen to the birds? A glass of water? Five minutes to dance to great music? If you can't do it now, make an appointment with yourself for later. (A bath perhaps).

Problematic Times of The Day and Find Ways

It is your life, and you are in charge, whether it feels that way or not. Being a victim doesn't help your children. Does bedtime drive you crazy? Make a plan to make it better, whether it's sharing more responsibilities with your spouse, getting started earlier, posting a schedule, getting more sleep yourself, or enjoying a cup of tea while reading to your child.

Immerse Yourself in Joy of Every Moment

Stop rushing and enjoy your child's laughter, the sweet scent of his hair, his joy in mastering something new. "Smelling the roses" fills your spirit. It makes life worth living. The fullness of your presence is what inspires your children to connect and collaborate.

Rules for Raising the Best Children

Parents often ask me which rules are essential for raising great kids. It seems that the most important rules for raising great kids are for us, not for our children. We start by taking responsibility for ourselves and end with a connection as the ultimate rule. Everything in between is about long-term coaching. The most important parenting skill:

Manage Yourself

Take care of yourself, so you don't let off steam to your child. Take action before your feelings get out of hand. Keep the cup full. The more you take care of yourself with compassion, the more love and compassion you will have for your child. Remember that your child will do every single thing you do, whether it's screaming or making scornful comments about your body.

Commitment

The most crucial parenting commitment is to be your child's advocate and not give up on him.

You Don't Scream

Appreciate who your child is and respond to what they need, not what you think they should need. Every child deserves at least one person who is 110% on his side. It does not mean that your child is always right. It means your child is always worth the extra effort; that every little love you put into your child makes a positive difference.

The Most Crucial Parental Secret

Punishment always makes your child's behavior worse. Avoiding it is the most important thing you can do to raise responsible and caring children. Instead of punishment, gently guide and set limits on behavior, but always try to empathize with feelings, including the feelings your child has about the limits you set for yourself. Both empathy and guidance/boundaries are essential; neither is successful alone.

Listening to Children

A safe place to express feelings while "listening." If you want to raise a child who can manage their behavior, they must first manage the emotions that drive that behavior. And if you want a child who can handle his emotions, he must first know that he has a safe place (your arms) to cry and get angry where he won't be silenced. Laughter releases the same tensions as tears, so playing with children is also a fantastic way to support them in expressing their fears and frustrations. Children who receive help with their big emotions when they are young learn to manage their feelings (and therefore, behavior) at an early age.

Expect age-appropriate behavior, not perfection, and keep your priorities clear. Your child is taking shape in front of your eyes, and he is still developing and will grow up, thanks to most of his inappropriate behavior. His messy room matters a lot less than how he treats his little brother.

Don't Take It Personally

Whatever your child does, it will be much easier for you to respond if you notice when you start getting primed. It's not about you; it's about your child, who is an immature human being doing his best to learn and grow, with your support. Cultivate a sense of humor. It will also help you avoid power struggles. Nobody wins a power struggle. Don't insist on being right; help them save face. When your buttons are pressed, use it as an opportunity to dig that button out, so it doesn't control you. It would help if you remembered when times get tough: All misbehavior stems from basic needs that are not being met. Satisfy their needs for sleep, nutrition, relaxation, pampering, connection, fun, craftsmanship, and safety. Let the children know in advance the behavior you expect. Give them "scaffolding" teaching, little by little, so that they can handle what is expected of them. Children want to be successful.

The Best Parenting Expert

Your Child. Let me show you what it needs from childhood. Listen to your heart. Be willing to change and grow and learn to enjoy the process.

Change Is the Constant

What worked yesterday won't work tomorrow, so your parenting approach needs to evolve as your kids do. Each of us seems to have the perfect child to learn everything we need to know. What matters most is to stay connected and never withdraw your love, not even for a moment.

The deeper reason children cooperate is that they love you and want to please you. Above all, safeguard your relationship with your child. It is your only lever for influencing your child. It is what your child needs most. And that closeness is what makes all the sacrifices of parenting count.

CHAPTER NO 3: POSITIVE PARENTING FOR AUTISM SPECTRUM DISORDER

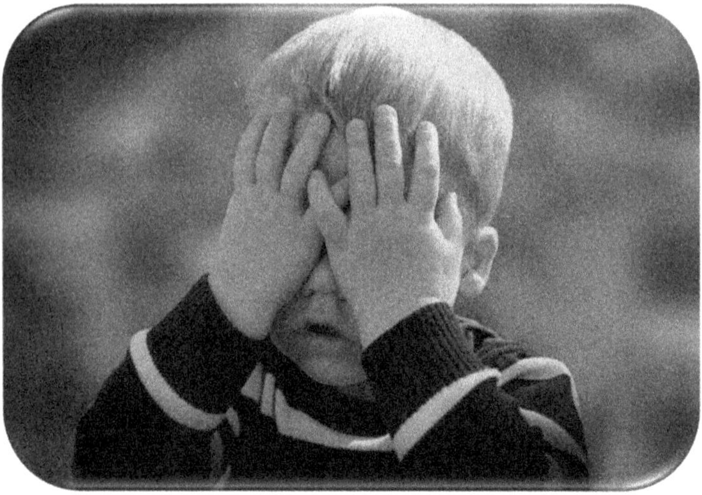

Being a parent doesn't mean how to discipline your kids effectively. It is mainly about cultivating their abilities, protecting them, understanding their feelings, and helping them deal with the world around them. We need to focus on how to help and teach them. The most effective way to learn is when you are loving, caring, and supportive. Someone who gives you positive feedback on how you are doing and helps you fix mistakes without being critical. For the first five years of life, your child is mainly learning from you.

You probably feel unsatisfied with how stressed you feel taking care of your preschooler. You are shouting more than you mean, you don't seem to like being with him because of the constant requests; he never seems to listen to you and does not do as he is told. It's time to improve the quality of your relationship. First, you need to remember what you love about him rather than thinking about the problems. Write a list of all the things you like and like about your child. He can be very affectionate, have nice curly blonde hair, love looking at books, be cuddly, have a good sense of humor, have a good, infectious laugh.

These are essential characteristics as they counteract all the problems you are facing, her hyperactivity, her tantrums, and her bedwetting. Despite problems, you love her. Unfortunately, problems can begin to overshadow the positives, and it's easy to lose sight of the child you love. You need to develop good qualities and improve your relationship with your child so that both of you enjoy being together. So, take time each day to be with him with no distractions or other work to do and no time pressures.

- Let him choose the activity and be there to witness what is playing, join in, and help." What a nice truck. Look how many cars you managed to put in the garage."

- Praise him: "This is a beautiful tower that you built. Talking about what he is doing and touching him positively, a pat on the head, and a quick hug that are not intrusive or demanding of affection."
- Try not to ask questions, criticize, give commands, or scold him during this time; be cheerful and attentive.

The particular time is for you to rebuild your relationship, to help your child feel special and feel that his or her needs are recognized. If you're not used to praising your child, he needs practice. It may seem false at first, but once you learn to notice the right things, it gets easier.

There can be a tremendous sense of joy and excitement in watching your child grow and develop. You quickly learn that your child is not a blank slate on which to write down your hopes and wishes for the future. He is an individual with his own needs to grow and learn, to investigate and explore. He wants to absorb the experiences of the world, and he needs you to modulate, protect, and help him cope with what happens. He is learning at a vast pace, but he thinks very differently from you. Many parents say, "It will be easier when he can talk, and I can reason with him," but in truth if your child wants to do what he wants, no reasoning will stop him. So, don't live in the false hope that it will get easier. He still won't listen to you. You're against willpower and a heady sense of success and power when it gets its way.

Sometimes they make mistakes and get into trouble, but it is a way for them to understand the rules and expectations of our complex world of adults. How many times have you been angry because your child's "exploration" went wrong? Is it someone's fault? As parents, we learn by trial and error not to leave out the markers when we are not around so that the background is not used as a sketch pad. Let's learn how to put locks on kitchen cabinets so that all the pots and pans aren't scattered all over the floor. Hopefully, as experienced and intelligent adults, we learn to anticipate events to avoid catastrophes. But do we do it? Do we become reactors to our son's behavior, waiting for him to do something that we then try to stop? Sometimes our children grow faster than we think and have moved on to the next stage of exploration while still going through the previous stage.

We want to encourage our children to be investigative, ask questions, and understand what's going on around them as it is a sign of intelligence. But we want them to investigate on our terms and in compliance with our rules. If they are not allowed to take Grandma's ornaments from her low shelf, you would say, "Don't, you will drop them and break them," or you would say, "Be careful, use two hands and then put them down gently. Can I help you?" it's a big difference between these two approaches. One controls the behavior and tries to stop it by blaming the child and anticipating a problem. The other helps the child explore safely with positive instructions on how to be careful. Help offers to alleviate one's sense of anxiety without upsetting the child. In one case, the child has learned not to behave. If he touches, he will drop it and break it; while in the other case, the child has learned a coping strategy, which is to use two hands and replace it gently. When this child goes to his grandmother again, what approach do you think will prevent him from touching the ornaments again, the one that stopped him and hindered his exploration, or the one that satisfied his exploratory desire?

Another big difference in these approaches is the involvement of the parent. In the first solution, the parent can shout from a distance and should not move unless the child obeys, while in the second solution, the parent is much more involved in thinking about the best way to help the child in that situation. Problem-solving takes place, and the parent has identified a safe way to explore the child. Usually, a parent in this situation goes to the child to avoid a disaster and help or show him how to keep him safe. Finally, we wonder which situation has the most significant potential for escalating child scolding? Tempers develop much more easily and quickly when an instruction is ignored. Telling a child to stop doing something tends to leave a void when the child has nothing to do, but saying a positive statement to the child about how to do it, or perhaps to do something else, bridges the gap and directs the child into acceptable behavior.

Myths About Autism Spectrum Disorder

Sad but true, this kind of misunderstanding still occurs in some places. However, as the number of people diagnosed increases to epidemic proportions, most people today have come across Autism Spectrum Disorder (Autism Spectrum Disorder). However, because Autism Spectrum Disorder is mysterious and has attributes that can be strange, awe-inspiring, and inexplicable, many myths abound.

There are certainly people with Autism Spectrum Disorder who are extraordinarily talented. Indeed, many may have untapped talents due to the challenges they face in communication, social relationships, or sensory overwhelm. Often what we see as an obsession is an indication of a talent that lies hidden and could be developed. Usually, those with autism have an inconsistent profile in which they excel or do well in one area and perform poorly in others.

Some people with Autism Spectrum Disorder are indeed geniuses, but not all are. Thomas Jefferson had features of Asperger's syndrome within modern diagnostic criteria. Others like Beethoven, Isaac Newton, and Einstein have all been mentioned as famous people who could have been diagnosed as being on the spectrum. However, for every person with Autism Spectrum Disorder, a genius, many others appear to be mere mortals like us. What is essential is to allow all individuals to discover hidden talents, or at least to reach their potential, whatever it is.

Due to the nature of Autism Spectrum Disorder, it is difficult to ascertain the cognitive level of people on the spectrum. Some or all of their senses are a hundred times more sensitive than others and therefore process the environment differently from neurotypicals (i.e., individuals considered "normal"). Second, it is increasingly recognized that many with autism have difficulty with "output"; that is, they can hear and understand what is being said (the "input") but are unable to respond verbally. Providing alternative means of communication can change the lives of many.

Finally, if you start with the perception that someone is not intelligent (considered "mentally retarded"), the expectations for that individual will not be very high. They will never be allowed to get as far as possible. Better to hope he's a genius and be disappointed than never giving a person the benefit of the doubt. Always assume competence.

If a person has one or two characteristics of Autism Spectrum Disorder, it doesn't necessarily mean they have Autism Spectrum Disorder. It is the number and severity of deficits in social communication and social interaction and limited repetitive patterns of behaviors, interests, or activities that cause concern. It is why it is essential to consult a doctor who is familiar with diagnosing Autism Spectrum Disorder. Many people are labeled "autism" (or "Asperger's syndrome"), who is bright and functional and doesn't need our help. Many of these people are responsible for inventions that improve our lives or artistic creations that make the world a more pleasant place to live. It is neurodiversity at its best.

What is Autism?

Autism is one of several related developmental disorders that are collectively referred to as Autism Spectrum Disorders. However, due to the difficulty in accurately diagnosing Autism Spectrum Disorders, it is difficult to determine what proportion of these children have autism. There has been a great deal of autism research, to date, and mostly focused on understanding the etiology of the disorder and seeking explanations.

The nature of the deficits that define it. It is now well established that autism has a genetic component, although the mechanism by which this works is not yet understood. However, it is suspected that several genes may act together to confer susceptibility. However, there may be several causes for autism, and indeed, the role of environmental factors in its etiology currently remains unclear.

In the absence of biological markers for the diagnosis of autism, diagnostic criteria focus on identifying a range of behavioral symptoms that are manifestations of qualitative impairments in the social, communicative, and imaginative development. The term "disability triad" was coined to describe these core areas of disability. There is a wide range in the expression of autism in individuals. There are commonalities in the symptoms shown of individuals to the underlying impairments. The impact of these symptoms and the significance of their families cannot be considered the same. In addition to the behavioral symptoms of autism, intellectual disability can also be evident. Still, again this varies from individual to individual in such a way that some children with autism may have profound intellectual deficit while others have "normal" intellectual abilities.

Autism as A Brain-Gut Connection

A possible connection between gastrointestinal dysfunction and autism was first hypothesized by Andrew Wakefield, a former British surgeon, and medical researcher, in an article based on twelve children published in the Lancet in 1998. In his article, Wakefield explained his hypothesis of a relationship between childhood gastrointestinal disorders and autism in those who received the MMR vaccine, typically given to children between twelve and fifteen months. Wakefield believed that the three vaccines (measles, mumps, rubella), when given together, could change the baby's immune system. It would allow the measles virus contained in the vaccine to enter the intestine, and some proteins leaking from the intestine could extend and damage the neurons of the brain.

Wakefield did not claim to have shown that the MMR vaccine caused autism, but this is what many have interpreted. The role of gastrointestinal dysfunction in patients with autism continues to be an essential research topic. Gastrointestinal problems can make a child's behavioral problems worse, and it's hard to do your best when you're in pain. More research is needed on the gut-brain connection. Still, parents of non-verbal children need to be aware that their children's behaviors may indicate underlying gastrointestinal problems that should be looked into.

Autism as A Neurodiversity

Around the same time that Wakefield's hypothesis was published, Judy Singer, an autism spectrum sociologist, invented a new word, "neurodiversity," to describe conditions such as autism, dyslexia, and 'ADHD. Singer's goal was to shift attention to atypical ways of thinking and to learn from deficits and impairments to diversity, convinced that many atypical forms of brain wiring also convey unusual abilities and attitudes. The word "neurodiversity" first appeared in print in a 1998 Atlantic article by journalist Harvey Blume. In the article, Blume compared neurodiversity to biodiversity, crucial for the advancement of the human race. The difference of opinion on autism brings to mind the Indian parable of the blind and the elephant. A group of blind people touches an elephant to understand what it is like. Everyone feels a different part, but only a part, like a leg or a tusk or a trunk. Each describes and names the elephant based on their experience of the part of the elephant they are playing. It is the nature of autism. The parent of a teenager, who is non-verbal, not toilet-trained, and experiences breakdowns will never be convinced that autism is just a brain difference to accept.

The parent of a child who looked perfectly healthy and then regressed at the age of two and has terrible gastrointestinal problems with constant daily bouts of diarrhea or constipation may consider autism a disease. On the other hand, the parent of a child with Asperger's independent and academically bright may see autism as a gift. The point is that they are all right, based on their experience.

The Future

Although we do not yet know the exact causes of autism, the past few decades have been encouraging for the wealth of knowledge gained. Since the mid-1990s, there have been tremendous advances in medical technology and science. The field of neuroscience has grown tremendously over the past decade, giving us a greater understanding of the brain, spinal cord, and networks of sensory nerve cells, or neurons, throughout the body, and how these relate to behavior, reasoning, and emotions. Everything necessary for understanding autism. We are learning more about genetic susceptibility, environmental triggers, the gut-brain connection, and the timing of exposure during periods of vulnerability for the developing nervous system. The growth of parent and professional-led Autism Spectrum Disorder organizations, coupled with ease of internet access, has ensured a potent lobbying force aimed at encouraging scientists and politicians to devote resources to research into the causes of Autism Spectrum Disorder and how to help the condition. There are many prominent scientists and professionals worldwide who have done a lot to improve our knowledge of Autism Spectrum Disorder and continue to do so. Over the past two decades, the number of nonprofit organizations dedicated to autism has increased dramatically.

Studies show that these children are often diagnosed later than their non-minority peers, misdiagnosed at a higher rate, labeled emotionally disturbed, and often over-treated. Many are denied insurance benefits, medical care, and treatment, directly impacting their prognosis. Although more research is needed, it is essential to note that the discovery of many successful treatments, therapies, and strategies was due to a strong collaboration between parents and medical professionals. Together they have formed a strong partnership, expanding the prism through which autism is seen and treated medically.

Why Seeks a Diagnosis?

If you have any concerns about your child, it is essential to consult a doctor experienced in evaluating Autism Spectrum Disorder. Hopefully, you have been unnecessarily worried. If not, you must have a diagnosis as soon as possible to access the services. Research shows that early and intensive treatment works best to help these children make sense of their world. Research shows that the sooner a child begins a course of treatment or therapy, the better the prognosis. However, research also shows that our brains have neuroplasticity, which means that it reorganizes itself by forming new neural connections throughout life. So, regardless of age, learning can still occur, and parents of older children should not be discouraged from trying different approaches to help their child. If you are an adult and think you are on the autism spectrum, just knowing that others like you can add an extra dimension to your life. There are now many adult-run nonprofits on the spectrum. These are great places to get information or join groups online and in-person to meet others who may have some of the same strengths and challenges that you experience. In the past, people were hesitant to apply a label because the "autism" label was permanent, and it meant there was no hope or future for that person. It shouldn't be that way anymore. Over the past two decades, there have been many improvements in autism with many new strategies and therapies available. Many children with autism can improve and even recover from any challenges that prevent them from living productive and happy lives. We are also learning to identify the strengths that many have on the autism spectrum and how to help each individual build their talents.

An Autism Spectrum Disorder diagnosis can open doors that would otherwise be closed. Your child may be eligible for early intervention services and therapies from local authorities, medical insurance treatment, and qualify for special education services. It will also allow the parent and practitioner to seek more knowledge on what to do, using the label as a starting point for collecting information. However, you must remember that you, as a parent or person with Autism Spectrum Disorder, own the label. It is up to you to use it or reveal it when it is useful or not to use it if you feel uncomfortable doing it or feel it is not useful or necessary. It's your information and your choice. Also, be aware that diagnostic criteria change over time and expert opinion on what those criteria should also differ. So, while a diagnosis is useful and necessary to access services, as a parent, you would be better off focusing on the behavioral characteristics that tell you the most about the child and how to help him rather than getting stuck on the diagnosis and what it means.

Characteristics of Autism Spectrum Disorder

Autism Spectrum Disorder is considered a neurodevelopmental disability, which means it affects the functioning of the brain. Autism typically appears during the first three years of life and is thought to be four times more prevalent in boys than in girls. While the past two decades have been encouraging in terms of treatments and research findings, over the next decade, we hope to learn more about autism as the technologies used in neuroimaging improve and understand more about the brain-genetic connection. The diagnostic processes of Autism Spectrum

Disorder are in a state of flux and are continually being improved as discoveries are made. What you have here is a street map of what is currently known and used. At this point, there is no medical test to diagnose Autism Spectrum Disorder. Any diagnosis is based on observable characteristics; that is, the behavior a person is exhibiting.

Due to the nature of the symptoms, Autism Spectrum Disorder is sometimes challenging to diagnose at an early age. If the child is the first, the parents have no experience to deal with. Seeing other toddlers and babies develop differently, they may start to worry. When expressing these concerns to relatives, friends, or neighbors, the parent will often hear things like, "It will grow out of it." Parents will sometimes talk to their doctor about their concerns about the child's lack of verbal communication and eye contact, his inability to respond to his name, and his obsessive attachment to specific objects.

In many cases, a baby will develop naturally and then begin to regress at around eighteen months. These children are generally easier to diagnose due to the apparent difference in past and present behaviors that parents and professionals can attest to by looking at photos, watching videos, and comparing observations. Some children have chronic ear infections; others may show allergic reactions. Many have intestinal problems: chronic diarrhea or chronic constipation. Or a child may have constant anger and/or sleepless nights. Parents can often be concerned because their child is a walking encyclopedia on a particular topic (such as trains), obsessively playing the same toy the same way, or only eating certain foods. Maybe it's the kindergarten teacher who notices that she doesn't seem to be engaging in conversation with her classmates and struggles with any changes in routine. Or a child may be considered "bad" at school because of certain behaviors, and perhaps the parents have not noticed anything wrong because he is an only child, or think that boys mature less quickly than girls. It may be accurate, but it's best to be safe and investigate your concerns.

The physician may hesitate to jump to any conclusions because not all reported observations are necessarily objective and may be interpreted differently. Everyone knows someone who talked late. On the other hand, a parent may not listen to concerns expressed by a childcare worker, teacher, or neighbor. It is unfortunate because of the earlier the diagnosis, the sooner the surgery, the better the prognosis. Some people with Autism Spectrum Disorder can reach adulthood without ever being diagnosed.

They may have always felt like they weren't on the same wavelength as others socially, emotionally, or sensorially.

Behavioral Characteristics of The Autism Spectrum Disorder

This list is not meant to be a diagnostic checklist but is intended to give you some ideas about the types of behaviors a person with autism may exhibit. Remember, it is the number and severity of these behaviors that can lead to interviews with a professional about performing a diagnostic evaluation. The damage to the state of social communication and interaction found in children were:

- As a child, he does not reach out to be held by his mother or seek cuddles
- He does not imitate others

- Use the adult as a means to obtain the desired object, without interacting with the adult as a person
- Does not develop age-appropriate peer relationships
- Lack of spontaneous sharing of interests with others
- Difficulty mixing with others
- He prefers to be alone
- He has detached ways
- Little or no eye contact
- Detached from the feelings of others
- It does not develop speech or develop an alternative method of communication such as pointing and gesturing
- He has the word, and then he loses it
- Repeat words or phrases instead of using everyday language
- Speak on very narrow topics

- Difficulty speaking abstract concepts lack or impairment of conversation skills
- Inappropriate attachment to objects
- Strange obsessive play with toys or objects (continuously aligns or turns)
- Dislikes change in routine or environment (furniture moved around the house)
- He will only eat certain foods
- Will only use the same item (same plate or cup, same clothes)
- Repetitive motor movements (rocking, hand flapping)
- Distinctive vocal characteristics (flat monotone or high pitch)
- It does not reach developmental milestones in a time frame or neurotypical sequence
- Low muscle tone
- Irregular fine and gross motor skills

- It covers the ears
- He doesn't respond to noise or name; he acts deaf
- It does not react to pain
- It becomes stiff when held, dislikes being touched
- Become hyperactive or unresponsive in noisy or very bright environments
- Eat or chew unusual things
- Puts objects up to smell them Often removes clothes
- Hitting or biting himself (hitting the head or slapping the thighs or chest)
- It spins like a top
- He has tantrums for no apparent reason, and it is difficult to calm down
- Hit or bite others
- Common sense is missing
- Doesn't seem to understand simple requests. Frequent diarrhea, upset stomach, or constipation

- Many of these behaviors are the person's responses to how they are processing their surroundings.

Diagnostic Criteria

With constant improvements in technology and advances in science, screening for autism at an early age is possible. However, there is no specific goal or medical evaluation that can be given to an infant, child, or adult to diagnose Autism Spectrum Disorder. Instead, several medical tests can rule out other conditions or help ascertain whether an individual may have autism.

Medical Tests

Medical tests are suggested to evaluate a child with autism, eliminating possible reasons for their behavior. Or to see if other specific disorders and developmental disabilities exist. The doctor you consult may also suggest other tests. Keep in mind that after a diagnosis, other assessments and evaluations will be needed to give you the information you need to form a treatment plan.

Development Screening

During routine visits of healthy children, developmental screening is a way to tell if children are learning the necessary skills when they should. During the developmental screening, the doctor observes and interacts with the child and asks questions of the parent. The doctor is trying to see how the child learns, speaks, behaves, and moves and whether the child has reached its developmental milestones or not. A delay in any area could be a sign of a problem. When such screening, or a parent, raises concerns about a child's development, the doctor should refer the child to a specialist in the developmental assessment and early intervention. These assessments should include hearing and lead exposure tests and an autism-specific screening tool, such as M-CHAT. Among these screening tools, there are many aimed at older children.

Magnetic Resonance Imaging (MRI)

The magnetic sensing equipment creates an image of the brain in excellent detail. Much progress continues to be made in this technology. At the time of this writing, MRI is not used to screen for autism, although some research indicates that MRI can show differences in the brain resulting from autism.

Electroencephalogram (EEG)

An EEG can detect tumors or other brain abnormalities. It also measures brain waves that can show seizure disorders. At the time of this writing, there is research indicating that EEGs may become a useful tool for detecting autism.

Genetic Tests

There is a genetic test that uses a cheek swab to examine infants and young children for sixty-five genetic markers associated with autism. This test was developed for use by families who already have a child with autism. However, at the time of writing this test, this test only identifies the estimated 10% of possible genetic markers. Technology is improving in this area.

Metabolic Screening

Laboratory blood and urine tests measure how a baby metabolizes food and its impact on growth and development. In particular, these should be considered when a child appears to regress, or other clinical evidence shows that there may be a problem.

Diagnostic and Statistical Manual of Mental Disorders

The DSM, the medical diagnostic manual, is used to identify and diagnose mental disorders and code insurance reimbursements. The professional who evaluates your child will make the diagnosis, or not, depending on the criteria specified in the DSM. The American Psychiatric Association (APA) released the latest version of the DSM, called DSM-V or DSM-5, in May 2013, after ten years of work on revising the criteria for the diagnosis and classification of mental disorders. In the DSM-V, changes were made to the criteria required for a diagnosis of Autism Spectrum Disorder. The new criteria are considered more thorough and rigorous than the old diagnostic criteria, according to the APA. Also, a reorganization of the criteria took place. In DSM-IV, the domains of autistic disorder included impairments in communication, social interaction, limited interests, and repetitive behaviors. In the DSM-V, the domains of communication and social interaction are combined into a single social / communication deficit. Additionally, a delay in language development is no longer a requirement for an Autism Spectrum Disorder diagnosis.

According to the DSM-IV definition of "autism," patients were diagnosed with four separate disorders: autistic disorder,

Asperger's disorder, childhood disintegrative disorder, or pervasive developmental disorder not otherwise specified. In the DSM-V, these separate disturbances do not exist. It has created some controversy between parents and professionals in the autism community, especially regarding the removal of Asperger's syndrome as a disorder. Those involved in rewriting the DSM-V definition believe that individuals diagnosed with one of four pervasive developmental disorders (PDDs) by DSM-IV should still meet the criteria for Autism Spectrum Disorder in DSM-V or another DSM- diagnosis. V more accurate.

In the DSM-V, the diagnostic criteria for Autism Spectrum Disorder are as follows:

1. Persistent deficits in social communication and social interaction in multiple contexts in the areas described below, which the individual

currently exhibits or has had in the past:

a. Deficits in socio-emotional reciprocity (for example, inability to carry on a conversation back and forth, inability to initiate or respond to social interaction, not having appropriate social approach behaviors).
b. Deficits in non-verbal communication behaviors used for social interactions (for example, abnormalities in eye contact and body language, lack of facial expressions).
c. Deficits in developing, maintaining, and understanding relationships (for example, difficulty adapting behavior to various contexts, difficulty

sharing imaginative games or making friends)

2. Limited and repetitive patterns of behavior, interests, activities, as demonstrated by two of the following, that the individual currently exhibits or has done in the past:
   a. Stereotyped or repetitive motor behaviors, objects, or language (for example, aligning toys, echolalia).
   b. Insistence on equality, inflexible adherence to routines, or ritualized verbal or non-verbal speech (for example, difficulties in transition times, insistence on the same food).
   c. Fixed and severely restricted interests are abnormal in intensity or focus (for example, intense preoccupation with or

attachment to unusual interests or objects).

d. Hyper or hyperreactivity to sensory inputs or unusual interest in the environment (for example, does not appear to feel extreme cold or heat, touch or smell objects excessively).

It is essential to recognize that to make a diagnosis of Autism Spectrum Disorder:

1. Symptoms must be present in the early development period.
2. Symptoms must be severe enough to cause clinically significant impairment in social, occupational, or other important areas of functioning.
3. Symptoms would not be better explained by intellectual disability or global developmental disability.

Comorbidities

A person can be diagnosed with Autism Spectrum Disorder and still have other existing medical or psychiatric conditions. In medical terms, "comorbidity" is the presence of one or more conditions along with the primary diagnosis. For example, an individual with a diagnosis of autism may very well have ADHD, anxiety disorders, and depressive disorders. If an individual with autism is non-verbal or has poor communication skills, observable signs, such as changes in eating and sleeping or increased challenging behaviors, should be considered as possible signs of depression or anxiety.

CHAPTER NO 4: PEOPLE WITH AUTISM SPECTRUM DISORDER

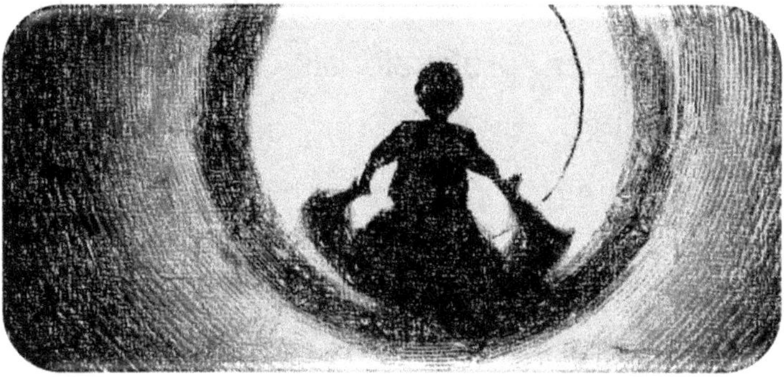

A diagnosis of Autism Spectrum Disorder is based on observable behavioral characteristics. We are beginning to understand why people have those observable characteristics, namely why they behave the way they do. From observation and written reports of people with Autism

Spectrum Disorder, we can understand what some behaviors mean. It is useful information for the general public to understand why people with Autism Spectrum Disorder might act a certain way, and understanding is close to tolerance! It is invaluable for parents, guardians, teachers, and other professionals to decide which therapies, treatments, and interventions might help a person with Autism Spectrum Disorder.

Behaviors Are A Form of Communication

For the very young and for those who are non-verbal, behaviors may be the only way for them to communicate with us and the only way for us to understand what is happening with them. Some of these behaviors are avoidance behaviors. Other behaviors indicate people trying to make sense of their surroundings or differences in movement, as explained above. Still, others are due to pain, anxiety, or panic attacks. The brain structure of many people with Autism Spectrum Disorder is different from ours. Some processing circuits wired differently, and it is essential to realize that they cannot help what they are doing; they are not just "difficult." Parents, guardians, and teachers can observe a person's behaviors and try to analyze why. There is a certain amount of guesswork involved, but by systematically choosing a behavior and noting your observations, you will likely find a pattern. For example, if a child keeps taking off their clothes, they are likely sensitive to the sensation of fabrics on their skin. It would be helpful to observe and take notes on this particular behavior, for example, if it does so when wearing a specific type of fabric or a precise fit or cut of clothing. Identifying what he can wear will make it easier for him to feel comfortable. Perhaps it can be desensitized by various sensory integration techniques known to be useful. However, the best way to understand what certain behaviors can mean or how to help is to read first-person accounts from those on the spectrum. There are books written by some severely affected nonverbal people and many by those who are more capable. We can understand our children more by reading what they have to say.

Discovering Balance Between Changing the Environment and Varying Behavior

As parents and guardians, we must find a balance between changing the environment and changing the individual. Usually, a little of both will be in order. For example, if behaviors indicate possible food allergies and tests indicate that this is the case, a change in diet (the environment) is needed. However, the person may need to learn to tolerate (slowly, through desensitization) eating certain foods they may not have eaten before eating on a special diet to alleviate their condition.

If a person has auditory and visual sensory processing difficulties, perhaps they can undergo hearing training or vision therapy and avoid spending too much time in noisy and bright environments. Classrooms should not be illuminated with fluorescent lights. Still, the child must also learn appropriate alternative behavior, such as requesting a break or permission to take a walk, rather than having a tantrum.

Listed below are some behaviors and what they can mean. Keep in mind that these are generalizations and that everyone is different, so they may not be right for everyone. However, this is a good starting point for trying to analyze a person's behaviors. So, looking at the treatments and therapies, you will already know the areas where you can help this person. Also, remember that some behaviors can indicate different causes, so you need to look at the person in general. Observable characteristics and what they might mean?

Selective Eating

- Eating only from certain food groups can be indicative of food allergies. Sometimes the discomfort created by food allergies can cause other behavioral symptoms similar to sensory processing problems. Frequent diarrhea or constipation often accompanies food problems due to allergies.

- Eating only foods of the same texture, smelling the food before eating it, and not eating foods that make a creaking sound can indicate sensory processing problems, as can chewing or eating unusual foods.
- Eating only the same foods, when accompanied by other examples of insistence on identity, can show a heightened sensory sensitivity or apprehension of the unknown.

Avoid Auditory Stimulation

- Covering the ears or appearing deaf (for example, not answering when the name is called) indicates difficulty hearing processing and high sensitivity to sound. A person can cover their ears to try to block out sound or tune in completely.

- Leaving a room when people enter can be a way to avoid excessive auditory stimulation.
- Listening to and repeating TV commercials or songs could indicate that the person has become accustomed to hearing those sounds; that is, he has become desensitized to them. Listening to people talking is more difficult because people don't usually say the same thing twice, and no two people talk the same way.
- People with autism often speak monotonously or have peculiar intonations because they don't understand the concept of nuance. The way you say something conveys additional meaning to what you say.

No Reaction, Or Strong Reaction, To Touch

Some children stiffen when you pick them up; some babies will fall and get hurt and won't cry. It usually indicates that their tactile sense is out of control. Maybe a child's touch sensors are overly sensitive, and they don't like being touched, or they are very dull and don't feel the sensations like most people.

Often Removes Clothes or Shoes

A person may not like the feeling of detailed textures on their skin. Some fabrics and shoes can make people with susceptible touch sensors uncomfortable.

Lack of Eye Contact

People with visual processing problems have a hard time looking at people directly; they usually look from the side of their eyes. Many on the spectrum have expressed that they can only use one sensory channel at a time. For example, they can process visually or audibly, but not both at the same time. If they want to process what the person is saying, they can't look them in the eye.

Unusual Body Movements

- Rocking in a chair, or back and forth from foot to foot, maybe a release of stress from too much or not enough stimulation.
- Touching your fingers could also be a stress reliever, but if you did it in front of your eyes, it could stimulate visual processing.
- Clumsy movements and encountering furniture can be symptoms of low body mapping, not knowing where you are in space, or low fine and gross motor skills.

- Difficulties with starting motion, stopping motion, or executing requests may be due to motion differences.

Lack of Interest

People with autism often lack the social skills and interests, which the rest of us find so important. Even a child with sensory processing problems will have a hard time being around other children who are, in their eyes, noisy and unpredictable, and who have textures and smells associated with them that the child with Autism Spectrum Disorder cannot tolerate.

Align Objects

- It can show the need for uniformity. Usually, the children who line up toys are also the ones who don't like change in their routine, can have repetitive speeches, and don't like to see furniture moved to a different pattern in their home.

- They may have a hard time making sense of their world. Thus, equality in specific areas provides predictability and security they lack in their existence that they are struggling to understand.

Temper Tantrums, Hyperactivity, And Self Aggression

- Keep in mind that all behavior is a form of communication. Trying to understand what the person is communicating is essential. Temper tantrums or temper tantrums in children can be a reaction to sensory overload or a change in inequality that provides security.

- Places with light and noise, like supermarkets and waiting rooms with fluorescent lighting, are difficult for people with sensory processing problems.
- Aggression towards others could be due to a variety of reasons, such as sensory overload. (for example, a sudden loud noise near someone's ear could cause them to jump to their feet and hit the person making the noise, as can be very painful), anxiety, or PTSD due to a past act of aggression towards the person on the spectrum.
- Self-aggression could be due to the search for sensory stimuli, the feeling of pain, anxiety, or frustration.
- Sudden changes in behavior can indicate possible mental or physical abuse of the person on the spectrum.

CHAPTER NO 5: AUTISM SPECTRUM DISORDER AND FAMILY

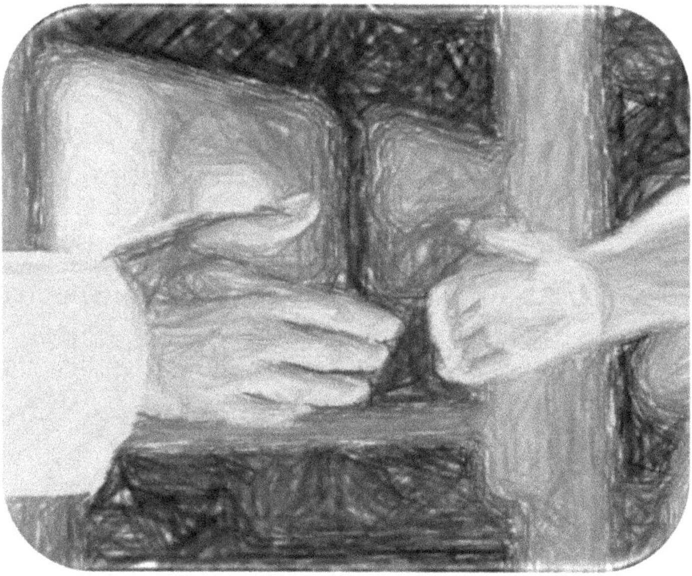

Having a child with Autism Spectrum Disorder has a major impact on the family. In addition to the stress associated with bringing up a child who needs more attention and care, children with autism are not as friendly as other children and do not approach their parents in the same way as other children. This lack of spontaneous signs of affection on one's child is very difficult for a parent. Families often tend to isolate themselves due to concern about their child's socially inappropriate behavior or fear of being embarrassed by certain behaviors of the child or the extreme fatigue that most parents of children with Autism Spectrum Disorder suffer. Families stop doing what they did before Autism Spectrum Disorder was very evident. Single-parent families find themselves alone with their hands full and with no free time to continue living any kind of social life, increasing their isolation. Being a single parent, adoptive parent, stepparent, custodial parent, or grandparent raising a child with Autism Spectrum Disorder adds even more difficulty to an already precarious situation.

A marriage or relationship with a significant person can deteriorate due to additional stress, fatigue, and differences of opinion about how to handle certain situations. Often one or both parents have a hard time coming to terms with having this child and are in different parts of the pain cycle. Add to that seeking support and trying to get proper education for the child, and it's easy to see how many couples end up getting it over with. Siblings may suffer from being raised in a family with a child who has Autism Spectrum Disorder. Not only do they have a brother who is difficult to understand, has limited interests, and is not social; they also have to do with some pretty wild behavior. They also feel the stress their parents are under and the fact that inevitably more of the parents' attention is occupied by the sibling with Autism Spectrum Disorder. However, research indicates that there are also positive aspects of having a sibling on the spectrum.

Extended family members, such as grandparents, also have difficulty dealing with Autism Spectrum Disorder. Some refuse to face the facts; others don't know what to say or what to do. Again, as a parent, it is up to you to decide when and what information to share. Much depends on the type of relationship you have with your relatives and how close you are to them. It is difficult to raise a child with Autism Spectrum Disorder. But first of all, you are raising a child, not a disability. No matter how serious the behavior or the situation, there is always a solution. And above all, it is the attitude of the parents that will make the biggest difference. This section offers practical tips on family life.

Children with Autism Spectrum Disorder

The sooner you realize that your home life will not resemble that of the Walton's, the better off you will be. Take heart from knowing that your family life would probably never be like that perfect ideal, and if it were, you'd be bored to death. Think about the Addams family and how much they seemed to have more fun regardless of the daily household disasters.

Life for your family will never be boring from now on. It might get monotonous, but it won't be boring. Start buying rubber gloves, cleaning fluids, disinfectants, and carpet stain removers in bulk quantities, as you will use them often. I wonder if the sales figures for cleaning materials are increasing at the same rate as the diagnoses of Autism Spectrum Disorder. But I'm digressing. It is not easy to find a balance between family life and inherent in having a child with Autism

Spectrum Disorder. It's true that you probably won't have the family life you imagined. But many people who don't have a child with Autism Spectrum Disorder don't either. People get divorced, lose a partner or a child. They grieve, but then they move on and rebuild another kind of family life. And families with a child with Autism Spectrum Disorder must do this too. Grieve the loss of your expectations for the family life you envisioned, and then start building what you will have. You owe it to the rest of the family. It will be hard work, but you can do it.

Don't Isolate Yourself and Your Child

First, parents need to ensure that the family is not isolated. It is vital for all members of your family. Now more than ever, you need to be surrounded by family and friends. Isolation occurs because you are too tired to go out, cannot handle your child in public, or are embarrassed by your child's behaviors. People soon stop inviting you, either because you previously declined invitations from them or because of your child's behavior or because you are obsessed with Autism Spectrum Disorder, and that's all you can talk about. You stop inviting people because you are too exhausted to be a hostess and are embarrassed by your child's behaviors. Don't be one of those people who say, "I remember when I had a social life. Look, I even have photos to prove it."

It Doesn't Matter What Others Think

Don't be intimidated by looks and comments when you go out in public and don't think you need to justify your actions to family and friends. If you are too embarrassed to take your child out in public, you need to analyze why you feel that way. If it is because of your child's behaviors, and they are very destructive or dangerous, then you need to work on those behaviors. If you feel uncomfortable that your child seems "weird," I suggest you get over it. Your child is here to stay and needs your support. And we must remind the general public that none of us are perfect.

Monitor Worst Behaviors of Child

It is never easy and can be extremely difficult at times. However, this baby is your responsibility now. You have to help him. First, you need to try to understand what is causing the behavior. If you can eliminate the cause, that's great. If not, you need to try to keep the disturbing behaviors under control. It's not fair to the rest of the family, nor will it make your friends in the community. There are positive behavior techniques that can be used to decrease and eventually eliminate worst behaviors, and with practice, a parent can learn to use them. Your pediatrician or local autism support groups should be able to provide you with a professional who can help you. If not, there are various books you can consult that will explain in simple terms what to do. They are listed in the Resources section at the end of this book.

Maintain Your Sense of Humor

Surround yourself with encouraging media. No matter how bad things are, you can do it, and you will do it today. Play good upbeat music, not songs that make you feel even more depressed. If you have ten minutes to read or watch TV, make sure it's fun. Don't waste it reading or watching the news. The news is usually bleak, and you can't help it.

Keep funny videos around the house and read. Humor helps, even if it's gallows humor. You may not control the situation you are in or solve your problems, but keeping your mood elevated will help you have a more positive frame of mind.

Do What You Can to Stay Healthy

Take care of your physical health. Try to eat right, catch up on sleep when you can, and exercise regularly. Even just a twenty-minute walk three times a week will keep your body healthier and make you feel better. Your physical health affects your mental health, which in turn affects the entire family.

Only Being Human

You can try to behave like a superhuman and do the impossible. Okay, if you feel up to it.

However, beware of burnout. Go back to being human and don't feel guilty just for doing what you can. Think about everything you have accomplished, not what you wish you had done.

How to Keep Doing the Family Activities You Enjoy

Most parents think family activities should be done as a unit. Parents of a child with Autism Spectrum Disorder can include the child on all family outings, hesitating to leave him at home while everyone else is enjoying themselves. Others may rarely take their baby out in public. What is needed is balance. Choose activities to share as a household that everyone enjoys, and plan other family activities or outings that can be enjoyed separately with individual family members.

Parents need to consider the activities they loved to do before and what they would like to continue doing now. See how you can fit them into the family life you have now. Analyze whether it is easier to change the activity or change your child's behaviors or leave the activity. You will probably have to do a little bit of everything. The following basic tips will help some of you, especially parents of young children and children with severe Autism Spectrum Disorder. These strategies are included here for those who don't have a supervised behavior program and need to teach their children some basic skills. If your child has a behavioral program, they are probably already learning these skills.

Basic Communication Teaching

The first skill your child should learn is how to communicate. Some children with Autism Spectrum Disorder are verbal and can communicate effectively; others may have enough words to satisfy their basic needs. Many do not speak in any way, or have spoken and then lost it. Not being able to communicate is very frustrating and can lead to great tantrums and disturbing behavior. Teaching some basic communication skills can alleviate much of this frustration. PECS is a wonderful way to help children communicate. At a basic level, teach the child that by giving you a picture of an object he wants, he will get that object. Without professional help, you can teach your child to give you or point to pictures representing what he wants or needs. It won't stop him from learning to speak and is a good, practical starting point to help you at home.

For example, start by cutting out the labels of the food or drink your child likes. When introducing this concept, get someone else to help. The first step is to pick a time when you know he wants a particular item. Make sure you have a photo of that item. Pick up the object and ask the other person to help the child give you the picture physically. In return, you can immediately give him the desired item. It will only work if he wants that item and can't reach it without your help. You can add more pictures, maybe laminate them, and put them in an easy place for the child to find, maybe pinned to the fridge or on the kitchen table. You can keep adding photos so that she can ask out, take a car ride, watch TV, listen to music.

Teach Your Child to Wait

Another skill your child will need to master to make home life easier is waiting. At home, he has to wait for someone to help him. He has to wait for dinner; he has to wait to go out. In the community, he needs to learn to wait at the doctor, wait at the supermarket checkout, queue to get on a bus or plane. Learning the waiting (you will eventually get what you want) will help reduce the number of tantrums. Here's how to teach the skill. Create or find an image that represents "expectation" for your child. We used a simple line drawing of a person sitting in a chair, with a clock face next to it. Write "wait" on the card. Laminate the image and place a piece of Velcro somewhere on it. Next, make sure you have photos of any items your child usually requests or wants immediately (favorite food, toy, car ride). The next time you request an item, put its image on the waiting card, then activate the timer for a few seconds. Say "We are waiting" or "Waiting" and point to the card. When the timer goes off, he immediately fulfills his request. Some children have to start with a wait of only three seconds and continue from there. Some may start at ten seconds or more. Once your child has learned to wait for those few seconds, add more. Know your child, so you'll need to consider where to start. Eventually, he will understand that he will get what he wants; it is only a matter of time.

Creating Programs

Another proven and reliable, useful method is planning. Posting pictures or words about the day's activities in the kitchen or at the front door can help a child who has a hard time making sense of the world around him. Knowing what will happen and in what order is comforting. You need to explain what the words and pictures mean verbally. Otherwise, children who learn with hearing may not make sense of the program. Many apps can help you with schedules on the go. Planning also helps those with sensory issues in some areas prepare for a not-so-pleasant sensory attack. For example, it is noticed that if a child is warned that he will go to the dentist or hairdresser, he seems to have an easier time, as if he has been mentally prepared. If the schedule is forgotten early in the day, and then show him the photo just before leaving the house, he seems to be anxious and unhappy, often refusing to get in the car, which he usually loves. If your child is very young and is at home all day, you may find it helpful to establish an activity routine that will fill part of their day and use a schedule to show what that routine is (eat, dress, play freely inside, doze, TV).

Be Consistent

For any behavioral changes you are trying to make with your child, you must follow it and be consistent and that other family members do too. If you introduce a way to communicate and then don't respond to his attempts to approach you, you will be doing your child a disservice. If you teach him to wait, but you don't give him the object he's waiting for, he won't learn the concept and be even more confused.

Family and Social Gatherings

While it is true that it is more difficult to attend family and social gatherings, it can be done. Meetings can be overwhelming, and attending with your child requires a certain amount of preparation on both sides, depending on the type and size of the meeting. It is a balancing act between making your child comfortable, making the other guests, and the host is comfortable, and making sure you will be invited to return. Your relatives and good friends may not understand why your child behaves that way, why he won't sit still, or why he is on a special diet. Some guidelines for managing family and social meetings:

- Prepare your relatives and friends for how your child might behave and what it means. For example, if your child immediately runs out of the room when there are more than a few people, explain that it is not personal, but that your child cannot tolerate the noise because his hearing is hypersensitive.
- Make sure they understand that your child is not misbehaving, but that you will keep an eye on him and teach him to control his behaviors, but it takes time.

- If any breakable items are lying around, you might ask if you can move them out of reach.
- Ask which rooms or areas are "off-limits" and be sure to enforce them.
- Just like a designated driver, you need a designated child observer. If you are going with another adult, decide who will keep an eye on your child and when.
- If your child is on a particular diet, you will need to bring some food that they are fond of. Depending on how well you know others and how they might react, you might ask not to leave out certain foods to munch on and bring something to share that everyone can enjoy.
- Familiarize your child with what will happen and who they will see, how to show pictures and talk about who will be there and the day's activity

schedule. If you anticipate noise, be sure to tell your child a couple of times in the days to come. If you know that some Christmas music will be playing, you can put it at home every day for a short time so that the baby can get used to it.

- Bring some familiar toys and favorite items to make the baby feel comfortable and more at home.

Travel and Vacation as A Family

Traveling can be difficult even at the best times when you have small children. Traveling with a child with Autism Spectrum Disorder can be even more difficult. Airports and train stations are areas that involve a lot of waiting. Leaving home safety for a new place can be daunting for a child with autism. How you prepare your child depends on his age and how Autism Spectrum Disorder affects him. Here are some tips that you can tailor to your child's needs and skill level. Remember that the first time you use it, it may not understand, but over time it will.

- Teach your child the "wait" skill if he doesn't have it.
- Prepare a monthly calendar and check each day until it's time to leave. Bring the calendar with you and mark the number of days in the new location, always indicating the departure date.
- Put together a "travel book" of images about the means of transport you will use to travel (plane, ship, train) who you will go to see (relatives, friends). Where they will sleep (hotel, grandmother's house) and what you will do or see at your destination (swimming, playing outdoors, visiting monuments). Repeat this with him as

many times as you like in preparation for the trip. If your child prefers a real book, a three-ring binder works best because you can add extra pages or insert the calendar above to use while traveling.

- Put together a picture or word plan of the actual trip to take with you on the trip. Add extra pages to your travel journal if you are using a binder to attach images or words in sequence. Add a blank envelope to insert the "done" images when you have finished that stage of the journey. For example, if you fly to Paris, start with a photo of the taxi or car that will take you to the airport. When you are at the airport, ask him to remove the taxi photo and put it in the envelope. Then have a photo of the airport, followed by the "waiting" photo, then on the plane, and so on.

- Think about your child's daily routine and the items they like or need, and take them with you to make them feel more comfortable. Bring whatever food and drink with you will make him happy on the trip.
- Buy small, inexpensive toys that he can play with. If you're only playing with a favorite item, try to find a duplicate and see if you can "break" it before the trip. Do not wash toys before you go, as your child may find comfort in the "home" smell of his special item.
- When staying in a hotel, it's a good idea to call ahead and ask for a quiet room. You could explain your child's behavior if there is a good chance, he will show it in the public part of the hotel. Same with a friend or relative's house.

- Make sure your child has an Identity Tag attached somewhere, with the current phone number and written "autism." You can order medical bracelets, necklaces, and tags to attach to shoelaces. If you can get your child to keep it in their pocket, also create an ID card with a current photo and date, as well as home and mobile numbers and where you are staying. Indicates that your child has autism. Be sure to add other important details: allergies, medications, and any specific information, such as if the child is non-verbal.

Talk About Other Problems at Home

There are other important areas parents may need to work on to make life easier at home. As you may have realized, it's not always easy to know how to interact with your child with autism to help you make a connection. There are areas where your child will need specific instructions. The ones listed here are important, but there are many others. Here are some suggestions:

Toilet Training

It can be difficult for some, easy for others. Some children who have sensory processing problems and poor muscle control may not "feel" when they need to urinate, or may not have the necessary motor control. It can take a long time to train some people.

Housework

Teaching a child to do chores not only gives them independence but also declares to the siblings that everyone contributes to the family.

Desensitizer

Some children with sensory processing problems have difficulty getting their hair cut, their teeth checked by the dentist, wearing a hat, and so on. Teaching a child to get used to an object or a sound, little by little, is helpful.

Behavior Plans

These are an important part of making life easier at home and teaching children responsibility for their actionns.

Social Skills Training

Children with Autism Spectrum Disorder must be taught social skills to participate in activities with other children. If your child is passionate about a particular topic or type of object, this could be a way to get them to interact with others.

Safety Training and Challenges

Many children with Autism Spectrum Disorder have no notion of safety, which must be taught to keep the child safe. You may need to make some changes to your home to keep it safe. Wandering and drowning are particular safety concerns associated with children with autism. Another safety concern is that people with developmental disabilities run a greater risk of mental, physical, and sexual abuse than their neurotypical peers.

Siblings Facing Autism

It's not always easy to be a brother, but having a brother or sister with Autism Spectrum Disorder has added challenges. These challenges can have both positive and negative effects on a sibling. Parents need to be aware of their sibling's feelings to develop supportive strategies to help them adapt. Some useful resources for siblings are listed in the Resources section. On the bright side, many siblings develop maturity and a sense of responsibility that are greater than their peers, take pride in the accomplishments of their brother or sister and develop a strong sense of loyalty. Siblings of children with Autism Spectrum Disorder are generally more tolerant of differences in people and show compassion for others with special needs. The downside is that many siblings resent the extra attention the child with autism receives, and some feel guilty about their good health. They may also feel burdened with what they perceive as parental expectations for high outcomes. Many siblings are anxious about how to interact with their brother or sister. There is often a feeling of resentment about having to deal with extra household chores, along with restrictions on social activities.

Living with A Brother or Sister with Autism Spectrum Disorder

Due to the behavioral characteristics inherent in autism, living with a brother or sister with Autism Spectrum Disorder is not easy. It's hard to foster a relationship with a sibling who shows no interest in being your playmate. After a while, the brother stops trying to interact with the brother or sister. It's hard to harbor tender feelings towards someone invading your personal space and snatching your favorite art project off the wall, or twirling its tail straight from one of your favorite stuffed animals. And how can a sibling feel comfortable, inviting friends, knowing that his older brother with Autism Spectrum Disorder could run down the stairs without clothes at any time? Some of the behaviors exhibited by children with Autism Spectrum Disorder would be typical of the behavior of a younger child. Still, it is difficult for a sibling as time goes by, and the behaviors continue to feel anything but resentment.

Sibling Concerns

Some of the concerns the siblings relate to Autism Spectrum Disorder itself. They wonder what autism is, if they can get it, and if their brother or sister will get better or not.

Many feel that parents spend more time with their brother or sister and therefore feel that the child with Autism Spectrum Disorder is loved more. They may resent the special treatment the other child receives and the extra burden and responsibility they feel. As they grow older, siblings are increasingly concerned about their friends' reactions.

How Parents Can Help A Sibling Adapt

Several factors affect how a sibling fits, including family size, the severity of the sibling's disability, the sibling's age at diagnosis, and the sibling's gender and age. They're placed in the order of birth. An older sister may feel responsible for a younger brother with Autism Spectrum Disorder and try to "mother" or take care of him. On the other hand, a younger brother may sometimes find himself caring for an older brother, contrary to the traditional roles he might observe in other families. It can lead to feelings of resentment. All in all, parents' attitudes and expectations have a strong influence on how a sibling adapts. A parent can do a lot to help a sibling adjust and have more positive than negative effects. Here are some suggestions:

- Keep the lines of communication open. Knowing that they can ask questions and talk about their feelings is the most important thing for siblings. Let them know their feelings are normal.
- Remind siblings that just because you spend more time and attention on your child with Autism Spectrum Disorder doesn't mean that you also give them more of your love. Let them know that you love them just as much and that they are just as important.

- Make sure siblings have a private, autism-free area to call their own. Install padlocks to make sure they have a safe place to store their valuable items. Siblings need to feel safe and have privacy.
- Determine the consequences for the child with Autism Spectrum Disorder if he destroys or spoils the siblings' belongings.
- Teach siblings how to play or interact with their brother, who has Autism Spectrum Disorder. When they learn the skills to get his attention and get a response from him, they will be able to interact with him on his level, and this will make them feel good about him.
- Regularly find time to spend with each of your children alone. It doesn't have to be a long time. A fifteen-minute breakfast alone can be beneficial for

parents and children. Plan a special outing now and then.

- Do what you can to try to control the behaviors of the child with Autism Spectrum Disorder.
- Ensure siblings can have friends and spend time with them without including the brother or sister with Autism Spectrum Disorder.
- It can be helpful for siblings to meet or talk to children in the same situation. Check with your local organizations to see if there is a sibling support group in your area. If not, see if there is any interest and start yours with other families.

For Your Child When You Are Gone

Thinking about what will happen to our children when we are gone is not always pleasant, and we would rather not have to think about it. But the reality is that no one lives forever, and provision must be made. No matter the child's ability or needs, there are always challenges you know they will face. If your child is still a small child or approaching middle age, a plan needs to be created. Many people procrastinate when it comes to this very important area for our children. Parents are so busy trying to cope with the present. Taking the first step towards realizing these plans recognizes that someday you won't be there, which's a painful thought. However, making plans empowers you because you are planting the seeds for your child's future, and you can rest assured that no matter what happens, you will have helped him as much as possible, even when you are gone. Would you like your child's future to be decided by strangers because you didn't make plans?

Steps for Planning Future Care

To prepare a plan, take a simple step by step procedure, without feeling overwhelmed by the process. Families are recommended to commit to knowing the following stages of life planning. If these steps are followed with the assistance of a qualified special needs planner, the family will create a comprehensive plan that addresses the lifestyle, legal requirements, government benefits, financial, and personal care needs. Regardless of age or severity of a disability, creating a plan is of paramount importance now.

Make A Life Plan

Decide what you want regarding residential needs, employment, education, social activities, medical and dental care, religion, and final dispositions.

Write Informative Directives

Put your hopes and wishes in a written document. Include information regarding health care professionals and careers, treating physicians, dentists, medicine, functioning skills, types of activities enjoyed daily living skills, rights, and values. Make a videotape during daily activities such as bathing, dressing, eating, and having fun. A commentary accompanying the video is also useful.

Decide on A Kind of Supervision

Guardianship and guardianship are legal assignments that require court-ordered warrants. Individuals or institutions manage the assets of people judged unable to go about their business. Guardians and conservators are also responsible for the care and decisions made on behalf of people who cannot take care of themselves. In some states, guardians assist individuals, and conservators manage people's assets. Many parents who have children with disabilities do not realize that when their children reach eighteen, the parents no longer have legal authority. They must petition the courts for appointment as legal guardian. Choose conservatives/guardians for today and tomorrow. Select capable people such as you to become unable to make decisions in the future.

Determine the Cost

Make a list of current and projected monthly expenses. Once this amount is established, decide on a reasonable return on your investment and calculate how much will be needed to provide enough funds to support your child's lifestyle. Don't forget to include disability income, social security, and so on.

Find Resources

Possible resources to fund your plan include government benefits, family assistance, inheritance, savings, life insurance, and investments.

Prepare Legal Documents

Choose a qualified attorney, paralegal, or certified legal document preparer to assist in preparing wills, trusts, powers of attorney, protections, living wills, and other necessary documents.

Consider A "Special Needs Trust."

A special needs trust holds assets for the benefit of people with disabilities and uses the income to provide for their additional needs. If drafted correctly, assets are not considered income, so people are not jeopardizing their Medicaid or supplemental security income. They also don't have to reimburse Medicaid for the services they receive. Appoint a trustee and successor trustees (individuals or corporate entities, such as banks). There are various types of special needs trusts. Make sure the person preparing your documents understands the differences and provides you with the right one.

Use A Life Plan Binder

Put all the documents in one binder and let the family/caregivers know where they can find them.

Review Your Plan

At least once a year, review and update the plan. Change legal documents as needed. Once you have decided to prepare a plan, find someone to help you or hire a professional planner. Referral sources are available through local government agencies, organizations, or support groups. Parents must do everything possible to help their children and as soon as possible. Some will be "recovered," and many will not. The goal should be to teach them how to make sense of the world and give them the tools to function to grow up to live independent and fulfilling lives. Helping your child learn by focusing on their area of strength or passion can make their life enjoyable and pave the way for them to connect with other people and possibly work in future years. As a parent, you may know, but you won't always be in control. You must learn to recognize what you can change and what you cannot. And this advice applies whether you're thinking about a behavior your child has or a policy your school district adheres to. In some cases, the only thing you may be able to change is your attitude.

CHAPTER NO 6: POSITIVE PARENTING WITH ATTENTION DEFICIT / HYPERACTIVITY DISORDER (AD / HD)

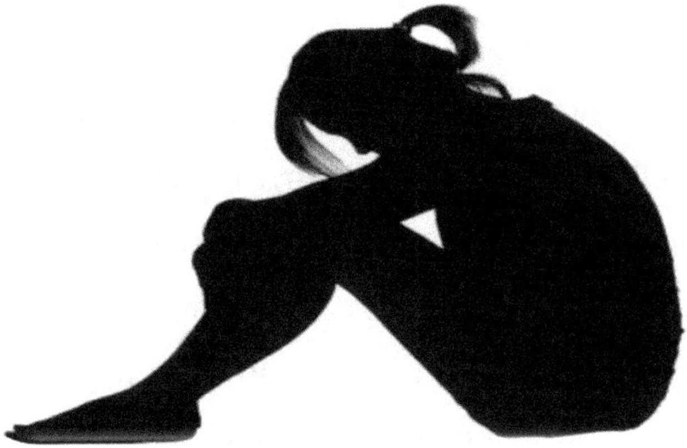

Attention-Deficit / Hyperactivity Deficit Disorder (ADHD) is the newest term given by psychiatrists to a childhood disorder with various names in the past. It was first called "hyperactivity," then "attention deficit disorder." The new term "official," Attention Deficit Hyperactivity Disorder (ADHD), was chosen by psychiatric experts. Although ADHD was described by doctors many years ago, its frequency has only recently been recognized. ADHD is often accompanied by learning disabilities in reading, spelling, or arithmetic, and also by other behavioral and emotional disorders. ADHD is more common in boys than in girls. Child psychiatrists believed that ADHD symptoms diminished and disappeared as children got older. Still, it is now recognized that ADHD is not a transient childhood disorder but is serious and can often last a lifetime, with symptoms persisting. Frequently in adolescence and adult life.

Along with a growing awareness of ADHD, a better understanding of its causes and treatment has developed. Although the behavioral problems that makeup ADHD and the academic problems associated with learning disabilities often occur together in the same person, it is helpful to view each disorder separately. First, not everyone with ADHD has the reading, spelling, or arithmetic problems you see in people with learning disabilities, and not everyone with learning disabilities has behavioral problems. Second, the treatment of ADHD behavioral problems and the treatment of learning disabilities are different. The following are the most important points are about ADHD:

- ADHD is the most common chronic (ongoing) psychiatric disorder of childhood. It is probably two to three times more common in boys than in girls.
- ADHD very often persists into adolescence and adulthood. Without

treatment, the child with ADHD is likely to have increasing difficulties in school. His non-ADHD classmate is much more likely to develop behavioral problems that can lead to "risky" behavior," at risk for himself and society, and therefore, in the extreme, in the eyes of the law. This behavior can continue into adulthood, leading to serious problems throughout adulthood.

- ADHD is not a recent discovery. A British doctor recognized the symptoms of ADHD in children, and the use of drugs to treat ADHD is also not new. A class of drugs called amphetamines was first used and still is available and is overall just as effective as the well-known drug Ritalin® (methylphenidate).
- ADHD is a brain disease that is probably transmitted by genes, which

means it is probably an inherited disease. It is not known exactly how it is transmitted, but it could be a difference in the structure or chemical functioning in the brain.

- ADHD often occurs with other disorders. The most common are learning and behavioral disorders, such as oppositional defiant disorder and conduct disorder.
- It is important to identify and treat ADHD in children as early as possible for two reasons. First, the treatment helps the child now. If the child learns more easily in school, it helps him avoid anxiety and depression associated with academic difficulties, unpopularity with other children, and conflicts with his parents. Second, early treatment can reduce the risks of problematic behavior. Children with ADHD are more

likely to develop in adolescence. However, children with ADHD have sometimes been described as energetic, "in a good mood," and creative. This disorder should not be viewed as an advantage or a "good thing to have." Rather, it carries with it a host of potentially serious and life-long problems that can fundamentally affect a person's life.

- The diagnosis of ADHD in children is made based on a careful history of the mother and father or others who helped raise the child. An interview with the child, and rating scales (used to describe the presence, frequency, and severity of symptoms) compiled by teachers and others who have worked with and know the child. Diagnosis of ADHD in adults is based on reports from the adult and a spouse or partner.

- There are no special psychological or laboratory tests to determine if a child has ADHD. As mentioned above, the diagnosis is based on the interviews described and on rating scales. Although no special psychological or laboratory tests can diagnose ADHD, there are tests to diagnose learning disabilities, IQ tests, and performance tests in reading, spelling, and math.
- In many cases, medications can reduce and sometimes eliminate many of the problems of ADHD in children, adolescents, and adults. An important point about medications used to treat ADHD is that they are not addictive in ADHD patients when taken in the prescribed doses. The second point is that the treatment controls the symptoms of ADHD, even if it doesn't cure it. It is not unusual in medicine.

- The psychological treatment of ADHD can be very helpful for children and, changes in child-rearing behavior can help parents cope with the child with ADHD. The educational remedy (special education) can help ADHD children who also have learning disabilities. Other psychological treatments show varied and uncertain promises, such as behavior therapy, with and without drugs.
- In adulthood, medications are effective and clinical experience suggests that couples therapy and psychoeducational therapy may be helpful. Other forms of treatment (such as group therapy) are being evaluated.

Characteristics of Children With ADHD

Many of the symptoms are present in all children and adults to some extent at some time. Consequently, parents tend to conclude that all of their children have ADHD. Before starting, therefore, we underline that the listed characteristics are not in themselves abnormal; they are abnormal only when they are excessive. What characterizes children with ADHD is the intensity, persistence, and pattern of these symptoms. Among the psychological and behavioral disorders is oppositional defiant disorder (ODD). Children are constantly angry, quarrelsome, stubborn, adult challenging, deliberately annoying, and even spiteful and vindictive. Even more serious is conduct disorder (CD), characterized by premature aggression, quarrels, truancy, lying, theft, and destruction of property. Numerous studies, often performed in clinics where schools and social agencies often refer children, have typically found a significantly higher frequency of both conditions. The list of characteristics presented here is intended to be comprehensive. It will include some traits that are present in some but not necessarily in all children with ADHD. Additionally, ADHD is three times more common in boys than girls, and girls typically, but not always, have less hyperactivity and fewer behavioral problems, and are less likely to have conduct and aggression disorders.

Attention Difficulty and Distractibility

One feature of the child with ADHD that is almost always present is an easy distraction or lack of attention span. This difficulty is not as obvious as hyperactivity but is of greater practical importance. The child with ADHD has no attachment. Young children, compared to adults, are relatively lacking in the ability to concentrate and complete long and boring tasks. The ADHD child behaves like a younger child. It is the opposite of someone sitting patiently in a corner, laboriously solving a puzzle, and tolerating no interruptions. As a toddler and kindergarten student, the child with ADHD quickly switches from activity to activity and then seems to lose things to do.

While the ADHD child may "only" have problems with inattention and distractibility, these symptoms "alone" can cause difficulties not only in school but also in his relationships with other children. The inattentive child may miss the point of a story that another child is telling and interrupting. He is therefore considered "out of it" by his peers. Or the child may lose instructions for a game and make mistakes.

At home, his mother notes that "he doesn't listen for long; he doesn't care, he doesn't remember." Parents have to hover over the child to get him to do what they want. Once he told him to eat with a fork and not with his hands, he obeys, but a few seconds later, he eats with his hands again. He can begin his homework as required but cannot complete them unless parents pester him. The child may not necessarily disobey the instructions, but during an assigned job, he starts doing something else. The tasks started are halfway through. His room was half-restored to order; the lawn is mowed in half. Sometimes, as discussed below, the child seems to remember but is reluctant to obey. At other times, he seems to be distracted by the task at hand and forgets.

It is important to note that distractibility does not always have to be present. Often when the child receives individual attention, he can participate well for a while. A psychologist may note that the child can pay attention during the test. A pediatrician may observe that the child was not distracted during the short outpatient examination. They are all correct, but what is important is not how the child can pay attention when an adult makes the best effort to get him to do so. Many children with ADHD can listen intently for at least a little while. If the examiner, child psychiatrist, pediatrician, or psychologist are unaware of the potential variability of this behavior, they may mistakenly conclude that the child is perfectly fine and that the parents and teacher are overreacting.

In some children with ADHD, distractibility may be hidden by the ability to continue doing a particular activity for an unusually long period. It is usually an activity they choose themselves. Sometimes it's socially useful (for example, reading), and sometimes it's not. The child may appear to "hook" and be inaudible or unusually persistent. The activity can be performed repeatedly over a long period. Such paradoxical behavior in a seemingly distracting child can confuse a parent, who will ask, "How can he be distracted when he plays his computer games for hours on end?" The highly unsatisfactory answer has to be: "We don't know, but that's it."

Hyperactivity

Not all children with ADHD are Hyperactive, and rather have problems primarily with inattention. However, most children with ADHD are very active, and when hyperactivity is present, it is very difficult to miss. Many children with ADHD have been overly active since early childhood. Parents often report that the child was "different" from the beginning of his life. Often, these babies are restless and have feeding problems and colic (intermittent and inexplicable crying). They also often have sleep problems of various kinds: some children fall asleep late and with difficulty, wake up frequently and get up early; others fall soundly asleep and are difficult to wake up.

When these children become small, many of them are bundles of energy. Parents often report that after an active and restless childhood, the baby stood up and walked at an early age. And then, like a King Kong baby, broke the bars of his crib and marched to destroy the house. He was always in motion, always in everything, always touching (and therefore, usually by mistake, breaking) every object in sight. When he wasn't observed, he somehow got to the top of the refrigerator or appeared in the middle of the street. In the blink of an eye, pots and pans were pulled out of the cupboards, and their contents spilled, glasses knocked off the tables and lamps knocked over. The mother usually thought, and with good reason, that taking her eyes off him for a moment was equivalent to causing disaster. The moment she turned her back, something had broken, or the baby's life was in danger. And he was right. Children with ADHD have more than their share of accidents, and children not with ADHD are much more likely to be seen in the emergency room. Once you have your driving license, you are at greater risk of suffering a car accident.

As the ADHD child grows, the description changes. He is incessantly in motion, driven like a motor, constantly fidgeting, drumming his fingers, dragging his feet. He does not stay long in any activity. He takes all of his toys off the shelf, plays with each of them for a moment, and then throws it away. Can't color for long. You can't read without losing interest quickly. He can't stop himself from struggling at the table; he may not even be able to sit still in front of the TV. In the car, it drives the other passengers crazy. He hits the people next to him, plays with the window switches, pulls the seat belts of others, and kicks the passengers in the front seat. His teacher reports that the child is restless, disturbing, unable to sit still, who gets up and goes around the classroom, talks, clowns, and who pushes, annoys his schoolmates. Sometimes the ADHD child is as talkative as he is hyperactive, chatting while moving.

It is important to point out that what is different in a child with ADHD is not their level of activity while playing. All babies make all adults look like sloths. The ADHD child cannot be distinguished on the playground. Its maximum speed is no greater than that of other children. What is so different about the child with ADHD is that when asked to turn off the engine, he cannot do it for a long time. Unlike other children, he cannot inhibit his activity at home or in the classroom. However, the child with ADHD doesn't have to be on the go all the time. Sometimes he can sit relatively still. Whatever the reason, this is more likely to happen when it receives individual attention from an adult. It is worth remembering because sometimes people who examine the child are misled when he sits more or less motionless for ten or fifteen minutes. They usually discover their mistake when they try to increase that time to an hour or so.

An important point about ADHD is that not all children with ADHD are hyperactive. There are children with ADHD who have many problems but are not hyperactive at all, and there are also some who are less active than normal. These children with ADHD are more likely to be neglected than those with hyperactive ADHD. The point is that obvious hyperactivity may be the first symptom to disappear as the baby grows. However, he may simply remain in a less obvious form. The ADHD adolescent or adult may continually fidget or stomp his foot and describe himself as restless, unable to sit still for long, and prefer energetic activities over quiet ones, other problems persist. Therefore, even though the once hyperactive child slowed down, not all problems were resolved. Many other problems may continue to require treatment, even if the hyperactivity itself has disappeared.

Impulsiveness

A very frequently described feature of children with ADHD is "impulsivity" or "poor impulse control." Every little child wants what he wants when he wants it. It acts without thinking or considering the consequences. The ability to tolerate delays, to count to ten, to think before acting tends to develop with age. Again, the child with ADHD behaves like a child several years younger than their chronological age. He quickly gets angry when things or people don't behave as he would like them to behave. Toys get kicked, brothers, sisters, and classmates tend to get hit when they're not doing what they're supposed to.

The ADHD child acts on the spur of the moment. He rushes into the street, onto the ledge, up the tree. As a result, she receives more than her share of cuts, bruises, abrasions, and trips to the emergency room. It is very prone to accidents. Wear clothes or destroy toys, not maliciously but without thinking twice. It seemed fun to walk down the street at its Sunday best; he wondered what would happen if he pulled that knob on the toy. Impulsiveness also manifests itself in poor planning and judgment. It is difficult to specify how much planning and judgment should be expected from children, but children with ADHD exhibit less of these qualities than seems age-appropriate.

Most children are more likely to run away in multiple directions at once. They are messy and disorganized. Their impulsiveness is combined with their distraction in producing messy rooms, sloppy clothes (unlined shirts, open zippers), unfinished homework, careless reading, and writing. Another area that is a problem in some children with ADHD is bladder and bowel control. When they are younger, some children with ADHD may get slightly wet or dirty during the day. They seem to pay no attention to their "urgent needs" and overflow a little. Bedwetting, which occurs in about 10 percent of all six-year-olds, appears to be at least three times more common in children with ADHD. It may be that bedwetting in some children with ADHD is related to unusually deep sleep, but that's not certain. It is important to recognize the relationship between ADHD and bedwetting because, in the past, "accidents" were often thought to be a sign of profound psychological problems. However, this doesn't seem to be the case. Often enuresis has always been present as a manifestation of ADHD and responds to the general treatment.

Social impulsivity, antisocial behavior, is sometimes a problem in children with ADHD. At some point, all children steal, all children lie, most children play with matches. As they get older, most children learn to inhibit these impulses. Some children with ADHD don't; they accept, lie, or light matches whenever they want. If repeated and severe, this can represent symptoms of a conduct disorder. Children steal for a variety of reasons. Theft may result from a simple desire to have or from a desire to have things that would acquire affection; it can be an attempt to gain status in a group; it can be a source of excitement, or it can be a means of revenge or to obtain attention or punishment. What is important is that if these reasons occur in the child with ADHD, he is less able than other children to control himself. It should go without saying that creating such a child would require a two-pronged approach: addressing specific motivation and reducing impulsivity (or increasing self-control). And, as with hyperactivity, impulsivity may not be present. The ADHD child may just be inattentive. It is important because, like hyperactivity, impulsivity is very noticeable while inattention may not be.

Attention Demanding Behavior

To develop normally, all children require the interest, involvement, and attention of adults. As they get older, they require less but still need the awareness and interest of those they love and respect. The ADHD child requires attention, but that in itself is not what makes him different. It is different and difficult due to its insatiability. As a younger child, he always wants to be center stage. He can whine, torment, tease, and annoy without stopping. Manifestations change with age. As a child, he may repeat annoying and forbidden activities; as an older child, he may try to monopolize the conversation at the table, play the clown in the classroom and show off to his friends at some risk and with the anguish of adults.

These aspects of his behavior may be hidden because he sometimes does not exhibit certain types of affectionate behavior. Many, though far from all, children with ADHD have been little demonstrative. In childhood, they weren't cuddly. They did not go to sleep on their laps but struggled to go about their business. They didn't get mad when their mothers left them with babysitters or in kindergarten. However, the same children have sometimes figuratively managed to stand at arm's length and prod their parents with a pole. The request for attention can be distressing, confusing, and irritating to parents. Because the baby requires so much, they feel they haven't given him what he needs. Because they can't figure out how to satisfy him, they feel moron. Finally, as the child can cling and strike simultaneously and endlessly, he feels angry.

Difficulty in Coordination

About half of children with ADHD exhibit various coordination difficulties, which, if severe, can be seen as a reflection of another condition, Developmental Coordination Disorder (DCD). Some children with ADHD have limited "fine motor control": they have problems coloring, cutting with scissors, tying their shoes, and buttoning. Handwriting is often terrible, and the child with ADHD perceives handwriting as a chore. The combination of poor coordination and lack of planning can lead to an illegibly written page with words beyond the lines, sides of the page, and each other. Others may have some mild difficulty with balance, for example, learning to ride a bicycle. Other children with ADHD may have poor hand-eye coordination - these children will be clumsy at throwing and catching a ball or playing baseball or tennis. Not all children with ADHD have these problems. Many are well-coordinated, and some are excellent athletes. When coordination problems are present, they usually cause boys more difficulty than girls because the athletic ability is an important source of acceptance by others for boys. However, even children with coordination disabilities may have no problems with activities that require large muscle groups and can run or swim without difficulty.

Resistant, Oppositional, and Domineer Social Behavior

Many hyperactive children exhibit interpersonal behaviors that have several distinct characteristics:

- A notable resistance to social demands, a resistance to "do" and "not do," to "should" and "should not"
- Greater independence

- Bullying behavior with other children

Probably the most disturbing feature of the behavior of children with ADHD, and the one most frequently responsible for their deferral for treatment, is the difficulty many of these children have in complying with the demands and prohibitions of parents. Some children with ADHD may seem almost impossible to discipline. In some respects, they seem to stay for two years. Parents describe them as "stubborn, negativistic, bullying, disobedient, brazen and indifferent." All discipline techniques seem fruitless: rewards, removal of privileges, physical punishment. "He wants his way. He never learns from his mistakes. You can't contact him. The punishment rolls off his back. It is almost immune to everything we do. "Children with ADHD differ, however, in how they exhibit resistance. Some seem to forget what they are told, while others seem to oppose what is asked of them actively.

As for independence, the child with ADHD is often overly independent but can be overly dependent in some cases. Independence can be noticed at an early age. The child with ADHD is the type who tends to wander ten blocks from home when he is two years old. When he is brought home by his terrified and distressed parents, he smiles and is excited. He doesn't seem to be upset by the separation. He is not the kind of child who is likely to be troubled the first few days of kindergarten or kindergarten or when he is left with his grandparents. The few children with ADHD at the other extreme, the ones who are overly dependent, tend to be immature, childish and attached. It is children who are most likely to exhibit the incessant attention-seeking behavior we have described.

The ADHD child's relationships with his brothers, sisters, and schoolmates are likely to follow a recognizable pattern. When he's younger, it tends to be a joke. Become proficient enough at catching other people's goats, annoying and annoying. As it grows, it shows a very marked tendency to be overbearing. Notice how this contrasts with his refusal to be ruled by adults. When he plays with other children, he strives to be the leader. He wants to decide which games will be played. He wants to decide what the rules are, and if the game isn't played the way he likes, he can stop.

Other children tend to avoid this, and, after a while, the child with ADHD is likely to be friendless. This lack of friendship is very different from what one sees in a shy and withdrawn child. The ADHD child is often socially bossy, and although he starts the friendship successfully, his style alienates other children. He will tell his parents that he is being talked about, rejected, and possibly even bullied. These reports are not excusing, and they are not inaccurate. They are correct assessments of what his behavior forces other children to do. "He makes friends easily but can't keep them." As a result, a child with ADHD often plays with younger children. However, a child with ADHD is not necessarily physically aggressive. He is not sadistic and does not like to hurt others. He tends to have more than his share of fights, but because of his impulsiveness and because brothers, sisters, and schoolmates are usually not thrilled to be pushed around and told what to do.

Emotional Difficulties

Many children with ADHD display some forms of emotional problems. The word emotional is one of those vague terms used by everyone in various ways whose meaning is unclear. Let's emphasize first that calling these emotional problems does not imply that they are psychologically caused. Indeed, most of them probably are not. Children with ADHD tend to have mood swings and periods, so their behavior tends to be unpredictable. They have great difficulty regulating their emotions. We all have good and bad days, and we can often connect our moods to our experiences. The child with ADHD is usually harder to find out why he was bad yesterday and good today.

Many children with ADHD are unusually unresponsive and hyperreactive. Sometimes they are numb to pain. They look unaffected and are less likely to react to the frequent bumps, drops, and scratches that are many of younger children. It is sometimes overshadowed by increased attention-seeking. When parents watch, they may tend to squeeze every last drop of sympathy obtainable. They are often relatively fearless. A combination of this fearlessness, craving for attention, impulsiveness, and a tendency not to "plan" tends to lead them into socially unapproved situations: as young people, in the treetops; when they are older, impressing their teenage peers with taboo behavior and soliciting the interest of the local police. Fortunately, such fearlessness is not seen in all children with ADHD. The over-reactivity of children with ADHD sometimes manifests itself in excessive arousal during enjoyable activities. Most young children will be excited at the circus, but children with ADHD tend to get quite over-excited under such circumstances. They may even lose control of themselves in less stimulating situations, such as during a visit to a supermarket.

This excessive reactivity can also be seen in excessive irritability or anger during frustrating activities. Of course, most children (and adults) don't tolerate frustration or disappointment very well. But the child with ADHD has a much lower tolerance for frustration and a more violent reaction to it. When things go wrong, he is prone to tantrums, tantrums, or dark spells. Many young children become irritable and childish when they are tired or hungry. An eight-year-old with ADHD may react to fatigue or hunger in the same way a normal four-year-old does. Although many parents describe their children with ADHD as "angry," what they usually seem to refer to is irritability and hot temper rather than aggression or hostility, i.e., hyperresponsiveness to minor comparative situations. "He's got a low boiling point, a short fuse. When he's angry, he loses control." Many children with ADHD are described as having good natures except during such outbursts. Another trait is seen in some children with ADHD that often disturbs parents could be called "Not satisfactory."

He never gets a kick out of anything, at least not for long. He can't be bothered to do much; nothing seems to please him; you can never satisfy him. This trait is sometimes produced by deterioration (children), but many children with ADHD behave this way without being spoiled. Their mothers may have noticed that they were unsatisfactory from early childhood. Finally, an "emotional" characteristic of most children with ADHD is also found in many children with other difficulties, low self-esteem. They have little self-confidence: "He doesn't think much of himself. He thinks he's bad. He thinks to be different."

Immaturity

Immaturity is neither a very scientific nor a very specific word, but it often accurately describes the behavior of children with ADHD. Their lack of social, athletic, and academic skills, their inability to remember, and to act, "do's and don'ts," are certainly characteristic of younger children. The inability to tolerate frustration (which often leads to tantrums) and lack of attachment are normal in younger children. Finally, some children with ADHD have another trait associated with immaturity, stiffness, and inability to tolerate change (such children, for example, will be upset if their routine is changed or if the furniture in their room is rearranged). From a practical standpoint, it is often helpful for parents to remember that emotionally, not intellectually, their child with ADHD can behave much like a child four or five years younger. Remembering this makes it easier for parents to manage their children. Parents don't know how to deal with a troubled nine-year-old but know how to deal with a normal four or five-year-old. If parents can remember that their nine-year-old with ADHD behaves in some respects like a normal five-year-old, they may find it easier to understand and help.

Changing Problems with Age

A salient aspect of a child's problems with ADHD is that they tend to change as they grow older. The behavioral problems that are evident in a child are very different from those in a teenager. There are several reasons for this. First, there appear to be changes associated with maturation; for example, the symptoms themselves tend to diminish with age (just as bedwetting disappears with age). Second, some changes occur due to learning: the child with ADHD is likely to be more hostile after his 10th year of peer rejection than after just one or two years of rejection. Third, the recognition of "problems" depends on one's understanding of behavior considered normal for particular age groups. Restless behavior is expected and tolerated in kindergarten children but not in second-grade children; reading difficulty is expected in all first-grade pupils, but it is seen in fourth grade. What is the usual sequence of difficulties? In infancy and childhood, the most obvious problems a child with ADHD has been in physiological function. They are likely to be irritable, restless, and have sleep disturbances such as difficulty falling asleep and frequent nocturnal awakenings. During the baby stage, his ability to do things increases immensely, and many of these are complicated things. The most disturbing traits are his constant "entering" into things and his inability to listen, that is, to respond to parental discipline. By the time she reaches preschool age, her attention and social adjustment issues claim the limelight. Her poor attention span, low frustration tolerance, and outbursts make prolonged play and participation in preschool difficult. Problems with her schoolmates soon appear teasing, domination, and other annoying behavior. These qualities endear her neither to her teacher nor to her peers. In some cases, lead her to the beginning of her academic career as a dropout from kindergarten. When she starts first grade, her restlessness draws attention: her teacher complains that she can't sit still, that she gets up and walks around, whistles, and drags. Academic problems, although often present, tend to be ignored. First, pupils shouldn't read immediately.

In some cases, it can include deception, stealth, defiance of authority, violation of social rules, and an inability to show consideration for the rights of others. It also often involves some degree of aggression, such as bullying and fighting, which can progress into clearly illegal activities such as theft, fire, and vandalism. Both the duration and the intensity of these problems are highly variable. If problems persist into early adolescence, antisocial problems, if any, typically become the center of attention. They can become more serious, including drug and alcohol problems, and even attract legal attention. If academic problems persist, they can now be taken for granted. It is not to say that the same child who has a reading problem develops antisocial problems. Rather, if the child has both reading and social problems, the social problems attract the most concern at this time.

Finally, many children with ADHD tend to overcome not only their hyperactivity but much of the other associated difficulties as well. Any child with ADHD can follow the listed developmental sequence and may no longer exhibit significant ADHD features at a later stage, say, as a preteen or adolescent. However, it is impossible to predict who will lose many or most of the symptoms of ADHD. The combination of problems found among children with ADHD makes up syndrome in medical terminology. A syndrome is a group of difficulties that tend to cluster, cluster, or move together. It is characteristic of medical syndromes for a given individual not to have all the problems associated with the syndrome. For example, some children with ADHD may have problems primarily with inattention and distractibility without the other symptoms we have discussed.

In contrast, most will have problems with inattention and distraction, along with many of the symptoms we have mentioned. These children who are not hyperactive are often overlooked because their behavior in school, such as daydreaming and staring into space, is not disturbing and is less likely to attract the attention of teachers and therefore go undiagnosed. It is unfortunate because these children are likely to fail in school and because they appear to respond to the same treatment that is so helpful for ADHD children with the additional symptoms described in the rest of this chapter. It is also important to note that the child who does not have some of the problems listed at a certain stage of their development is very unlikely to develop them at a later stage. The child who does not have coordination problems when he is young will not have them when he is older. The child who has no reading problems when he is seven or eight will not have them as a teenager. For parents living with those difficulties their ADHD child has, this positive aspect of their development can comfort. It is not understated, as observed by doctors who have treated these children and worked with their families for periods of years. Therefore, although ADHD is a lifelong phenomenon, in many cases, its symptoms gradually subside and become of little consequence as a person ages into adulthood. The most likely symptom that "almost" disappears is hyperactivity.

Oppositional Defiant Disorder and Conduct Disorder

Of the various conditions that can occur alongside ADHD, perhaps the most troubling is Oppositional Defiant Disorder (ODD) and Conduct Disorder (CD). These are both more likely in boys, in children with significant hyperactivity, and in children who show early aggression. The more severe the early symptoms of ADHD and the more prominent the early antisocial behavior, the more likely the child will develop one or both disorders and the disease. The ADHD child who transforms resistant behavior into defiant behavior is classified as suffering from ODD. This disorder is described as a "recurring pattern of negativistic, provocative, disobedient, and hostile behavior towards authoritarian figures." He often loses his temper, argues with adults, actively defies their requests, deliberately does things to annoy others, and is angry and resentful or spiteful and vindictive. This behavior is very difficult for parents and teachers to deal with. Equally important, the child with ODD has a higher risk of developing CD.

The main problem of CD children is "a repetitive and persistent pattern of behavior in which the fundamental rights of others or the main norms or rules of society are violated." Such children are aggressive, threaten and intimidate others, engage in physical fights, can be physically cruel to people or animals, destructive to property (including fire), lie, steal, drift, and grossly violate the rules of family and society. In particularly severe cases, the child may show numbness and a lack of remorse or guilt. About half of CD children continue to behave like adults and often have confrontations with the police and spend time in prison. ADHD with CD is more severe than ADHD alone, and most doctors believe it should be treated vigorously at an early age. Other disorders may be present in ADHD children, such as anxiety disorders, severe depression, and bipolar disorder. Still, it is unclear whether there is a higher frequency of these disorders among ADHD children.

CHAPTER NO 7: UNDERSTAND AND ADDRESS THE PROBLEM ADHD

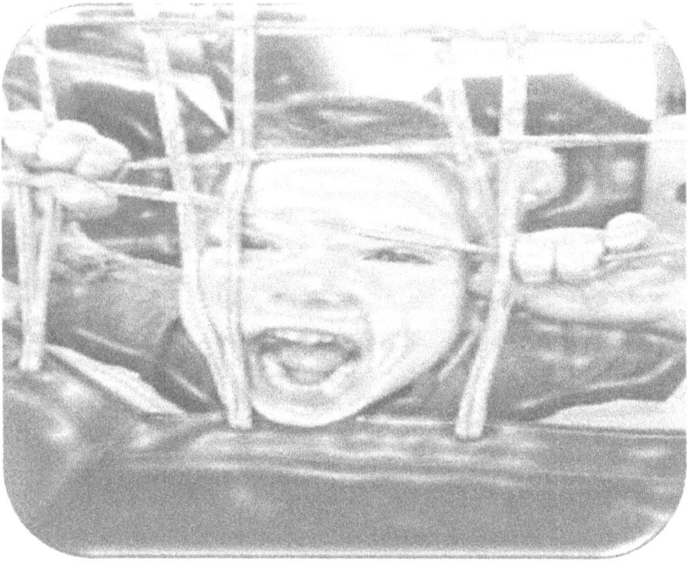

How should a parent handle problem? It seems that if a problem is psychological, the child is responsible for its behavior. If it's good, it should be praised, and if it's bad, it should be punished. Similarly, if the problem is physical, the child is not responsible for his behavior. If so, he shouldn't be rewarded for being good or punished for being bad. None of these beliefs are true. Temperament can influence behavior, but it is not the only factor that determines behavior. Temperament can make it easier or harder for a child to control himself. It may make it easier for him to learn to respond to discipline. But the way parents feel about the child, and the way they treat him can have appreciable effects. In recent years, psychiatrists and psychologists have found that patients whose severe psychological problems are physically caused can benefit greatly from certain psychological techniques. These techniques are based on three principles:

1. Making patients accountable for their behavior
2. Reward them for good behavior
3. Punish them (especially) for misconduct

The child with ADHD does best when held accountable and accountable for their behavior. He shouldn't be allowed to say, either in so many words or indirectly, "I'm ADHD, I'm a mental cripple, I'm not responsible for what I do." He should be treated as responsible and, if necessary, be told something to that effect: "You have problems that can sometimes make it difficult for you to control yourself. But the same is true for everyone. Everyone does some things easier than others and does other things with more difficulty. You can learn to (count to ten, stay calm), and it is expected you to. As with all of our suggestions, of course, parents should change the words to suit them and their parents.

The child should not be found irresponsible or blameworthy but should be treated as someone who has a greater than average tendency to have certain types of difficulties. Parents should realize that for most children with ADHD, no rearing method will eliminate the core symptoms of ADHD. The child will tend to be more alert and forgetful and will seem distracted and stubborn, regardless of parental discipline. In most cases, it doesn't do these things to annoy. He would have performed them regardless of how he was raised. Parents should make a clear distinction between symptoms that can be benefited by both parenting and medicine and those that can only be alleviated by medicine. It will prevent parents from using psychological methods to change things that cannot change in this way. These psychologically immutable symptoms usually include the following: short attention span, distraction, moodiness, lack of attachment, poor academic performance, and immaturity. They can include bedwetting, dirt, and some antisocial behaviors like theft. Although psychological techniques generally do not eliminate these problems in the child, they can change them. For example, the child may continue to have tantrums, but he can be taught what to do when he has them.

In summary, parents need to remember three things. One, the child has difficulty doing and not doing certain things. Second, he will learn better how to compensate for his problems if he is treated as a responsible person who can gradually learn to control himself and his behavior. Three, the degree to which particular child-rearing techniques can help his problems varies. It is much easier to teach him how to control his temper or take responsibility for his chores than to teach him to have a longer attention span or be less distracting. Both medicine and discipline will help the first type of problems (for example, temperament and housework). The second type of problem (for example, short attention span), for the most part, can only be solved by medicine. The main problem of the child with ADHD at home relates to discipline. By discussing the basic procedures that will help the child function effectively in their family environment, we will first indicate how parents can establish constructive rules. The second section will describe the rewards and punishments most likely to ensure that the child will adhere to these results.

Establish Rules

There is considerable evidence that certain ways of treating children with ADHD are more effective than others. A solid, consistent, explicit, and predictable home environment is best. Let me elaborate on the special meaning these terms have concerning the discipline of the child with ADHD. Stationary means that the rules or expectations for the child always have the same consequences. If he breaks a particular rule, he is always punished and always in the same way. If he does what is asked of him, he always gets recognition or praise. Consistency means the rules themselves don't change every day. If he has to clean his room before he goes to play, he is never allowed to leave his room until it has been cleaned. Explicit means clearly defined and clearly understood by all parties. For example, "cleaned" could mean clothes have been hung in the closet, toys have been put back on a shelf, or the room has been vacuumed and dusted any combination. For the cleanliness rule, the definition of cleanliness must be explicit enough so that the child and parents understand the rule equally. Predictable means that the laws are made before, not after the crime.

Of course, all the parent's expectations for the child cannot be stated in advance. Parents never think of telling the child not to put nail polish on the carpet, and they rarely think of telling him not to put a toy car in his ear. Some things can only be fixed after they have happened. In general, however, for most daily activities, rules can and should be established and then enforced. The child has to wash, brush his teeth, do housework, and homework every day; rules should be established regarding these routine functions. Applying these rules should follow any violations, such as removing them from the environment or removing things that distract them, but should not be employed if the rules have not been agreed in advance. Similar consistent and predictable rules for adults exist within speed limits for driving. It is easier to adhere to a specific speed limit, say 55 mph than to adhere to the vague, "reasonable and correct" limit previously designated in some Western states. In the vague speed limit, it is unknown how fast you can go if it is dusk, and light rain is falling.

These tips can impress parents as tough and possibly cruel. They may also appear to contradict various benign permissive doctrines that advocate allowing children to "do their own thing" and allowing parents and children to discuss things. Let's try to correct some common misconceptions. First, firmness is not the same as hardness. Harshness is an overly strict or brutal application of the rules. It is adamant about finding him every time he does so. Second, children need structure. They need established rules, expectations, and values by which to live. This structure does not mean the absence of freedom.

Firm and consistent rules of conduct have nothing to do with the child's self-expression or understanding between parent and child. We talked about rules of behavior, not rules for thoughts and feelings. Thoughts and feelings are very different from behavior. They cannot be regulated, and the parent should not attempt to regulate them. As discussed, parents should help their children recognize and express their feelings. But both parents and children should always discriminate between feelings and behaviors. For example, parents of a child with ADHD should allow him to express his feelings of jealousy towards his newborn sister, but he should not be allowed to beat her. Feeling jealous and hitting because of jealousy should be recognized as being as different as night and day.

Finally, the definition of firm rules must not interfere with useful discussions between the parents and the child. As the child grows, such discussions should certainly be a part of family life, but even when younger, they can be helpful. The child may, for example, suggest ways to do his homework in a way that he likes best, and that doesn't compromise the family. It is perfectly acceptable and should be encouraged. But talking about things shouldn't prevent rules from being formulated. It can affect how they are decided, and it can change their exact terms, but it shouldn't interfere with their explicit and consistent definition. What specific rules should be in a particular family depend on the preferences of the parents and the age of the child? Parents could theoretically set rules and teach children to respect them. (Different cultures have very different rules and standards for children's behavior, and each culture tries to create a "standard product," a child well adapted to living in that culture.) As the child grows, the freedom of parents 'setting these rules decreases. The young child is mostly only aware of how his or her family does things. The older child is very aware of how other children and their families do things and will tend to rebel if their standards appear different.

Rewards and Punishments

In addition to establishing solid rules to help the child, parents must predetermine a reward and punishment plan. These rewards and punishments should be seen as such by the child and not just by the parents. The words "reward" and "punishment" have an unfortunate meaning for some people. "Prize" seems to suggest corruption and "punishment" to suggest brutality. All that is meant by reward is something the child likes, especially attention, praise, or a little special privilege. Some privileges, toys, and so on can be useful under special conditions, which will be discussed later. Likewise, punishment simply means something the child doesn't like. It does not mean beatings, emotional abandonment, or denial of privileges for a long time. In general, with younger children, a more effective and painless punishment is to use "timeout," such as sending the child to his room until he stops acting unwanted (for example, throwing a tantrum) or ends a required task (for example, dressing). It is more effective to say, "Go to your room, please, and come back for breakfast when your shoes are fastened, and your face is washed," rather than yelling at the baby or spanking him.

There are two other important principles of reward and punishment. First, to be extremely useful, a reward or punishment should be immediate. Any delay decreases effectiveness. When a child does what you want him to do, praise him right away. If he does what he was told not to do, punish him immediately. Don't give away gifts (any toy you want in two weeks) or threaten punishment (Father will spank you when he gets home). Second, a one-off rule should be adopted. Parents should learn the habit of saying do or not do only once before rewarding or punishing. If they don't apply this rule, if they give the first, second, third, and tenth warning before taking action, their children will learn to commit ten violations before they worry.

Meanwhile, the parents will have developed a sore throat and built up a good deal of anger. In some cases, the child may have anxiously pushed his parents to take sides. Surprisingly, most children feel relieved when the parent finally takes action. You can avoid a good deal of friction by using this unique rule. What strengthens children? It depends on their state. For the rat that has eaten their fill, the food will no longer strengthen and will not lower a bar to get it. For a thirsty child, water can be strengthening; for a hungry child, food can be strengthening. However, most of the child's acts are influenced by the behavior of the parents, which is very different from the mere satisfaction of hunger or thirst. For a single child, reinforcing behavior varies, but some parental acts and behaviors are reinforcing for nearly all children. The most important, as we have suggested, is the affection of the parents and the attention of the parents. Parental attention is probably the single most common reinforcement in a child's daily life. It is important not only because of how often it is focused on the child but also because it strengthens itself regardless of what arouses it. Some types of punishment, therefore, are more rewarding for a child than ignoring them. Expressing disapproval of a child's most recent misdeed is giving him attention.

Some punishments focus attention on the child and thereby reinforce misconduct. If severe, punishment is likely to produce negative side effects; therefore, the question arises as to whether any form of punishment can be reasonably effective. Although psychologists disagree, there appear to be lesser degrees of punishment that can suppress the behavior but only temporarily. Shocks that do not make the animal neurotic will probably not be effective for a long time.

The relevance of this to children should be pretty obvious. Human parents use only moderate punishment. Children with ADHD, who are often not particularly sensitive to punishment, the effects of punishment should not be expected to be long-lasting. And indeed, they rarely are.

Positive reinforcement, on the other hand, may not even be permanent, but with some tweaks, it can be extremely long-lasting. Its virtue is that once the child starts on the right path, he is likely to receive reinforcement from people outside the family. The child who is taught to be reasonably educated and in whom drugs help to be moderately obedient and reasonably non-aggressive will be strengthened by the favorable attention of others, making friends, and succeeding.

The Management of The Common Problems of The ADHD Child

The procedures, principles, and techniques described so far refer to general approaches to the child with ADHD. Also, we have some special tips that can help you deal with some common problems specific to these children.

Get the Child's Attention

One of the biggest problems a child with ADHD has is paying attention. And one of the main problems of the parent of a child with ADHD is getting the child's attention. If you want to communicate effectively with a child with ADHD, you need to use some special techniques. For example, often, the parent will give a command or request to a preschooler with ADHD while the child's attention is elsewhere. In children without ADHD, this request from the parent can draw the child's attention. In the case of the ADHD child, it usually doesn't. Even if the parent has the attention of the child with ADHD, the child may not want to hear what the parent has to say and may put his hands on his ears or turn his head away. The following procedure should, therefore, be employed: The parent should gently take the head (or shoulders) of the child with ADHD in their hands and give the child the message. To ensure that the child has received the message, the parent should ask the child what they were told, not in a punitive way but a neutral tone. If the child does not know, the parent should make the statement again. Physical contact appears to play an important role in getting the child's attention. When the message is given with the parent's hands resting on the baby's shoulders, the baby appears to pay more attention than it does when not being touched.

Rigidity

A feature of some children with ADHD, although it can also be seen in Non-ADHD children, is stiffness. Stiff children get angry when their activities are interrupted, or their routine is changed. For example, they can become furious if they are prevented from playing with their toys so they can be taken to visit their grandmother. Or they may start screaming if the order to wear the clothes is varied. A three-year-old boy with ADHD had a quirk if the family went to his grandmother's house for a different route. Stiffness sometimes subsides with age, but effective ways to deal with it before that blessed time comes. The main principle is anticipation. Long before the break in the routine occurs, the parent should repeatedly tell the child what is about to happen. Even before the child can read the time, they can recognize when the pointer approaches, setting the bell to ring. Instead of counting down every morning to get dressed for school, the timer can be replaced.

Similarly, considerable pain can often be avoided by discussing long-term changes before they occur. Repeated anticipatory speeches on issues such as moving furniture, new sleeping arrangements, and modified school schedules can often lessen the shock to the stiff child. These procedures, of course, do not change the stiffness of the child, but they lessen its unpleasant impact.

Dizzying Loss of Control

A very common problem of children with ADHD, both in preschool and in the first elementary school, is a dizzying loss of behavioral control. It refers to the fact that the child is becoming wilder and behaving more and more immature once he is gone.

For example, when guests arrive, the child may behave in a way that seeks attention, and, as soon as he receives attention, he may react with silly and noisy behaviors that constantly worsen. After first telling guests a story or showing some of his models, he may start talking louder, start running around, and in some cases, bounce off walls. It can also happen in noisy or stimulating situations, such as the supermarket or the circus.

How can this loss of control be managed? It is helpful for parents to learn to recognize the early symptoms of this behavioral burnout. It is much easier to reverse such cycles soon after they start than in full swing. When parents recognize the symptoms of an impending behavioral spiral, they should warn the child with a phrase that is always used when the child is aroused - and here we again see the tagging technique in action.

Different parents use different phrases. Some parents will say, "You're getting too wild," while others may warn, "You're getting over-excited."

The important point is to label the same type of behavior the same way every time so that the child can learn what the parents mean by the special phrase. After the parents identify the behavior, the child should be told to go to his room and stay there until he calms down. If necessary, he should be taken to his room. Once he has calmed down, the child should not receive any punishment but should receive praise for taking control of himself and acting like a big boy. Then, in a non-accusatory tone of voice, the parent should explain to the child what happened before and what prompted the parent to label that behavior as wild or over-excited. In other words, parents should make sure the child is praised for behaving adult enough and that the child does not receive any extra attention, positive or negative, for being out of control. Therefore, the best thing to do against spiraling loss of control is to try to avoid it. To use a variation on an old cliché, parents should be ready with that invaluable ounce of prevention. They should learn to recognize the situations that trigger these spiral reactions and avoid them or move the child away from them as soon as possible.

Verbal Tantrums

One of the types of loss of control seen in both younger and older children with ADHD is a verbal tantrum. Such behavior is probably more mature than the spells of holding their breath or kicking the floor, but parents are not thrilled with this type of maturation. During tantrums, the child may speak (or scream) continuously, criticizing, blaming others, and denying responsibility. It can raise not only trivial issues but honesty issues that exist in the family. These uninterrupted productions are limited only by his talkativeness and the way his parents handle the problem. Most parents' natural reaction is to argue. The main advice we have is that a parent shouldn't argue at all. A screaming mutual encounter solves nothing. While the child has tantrums, he should be told that things will be discussed when he calms down. If he cannot calm down, he should be placed in a suspension room, and only after calming down should the parent talk to the child about the real problem. Parents who often find themselves screaming can take this as a warning sign that they are doing something wrong, not bad, just ineffective.

Make the Child Responsible

All parents hope that the child will eventually take responsibility for monitoring their behavior. The procedure discussed in "Household Chores" illustrates one way to establish a habit of responsibility. Here we will describe another method of encouraging accountability. This example deals with another recurring problem for children with ADHD, forgetting to take homework home, which means they don't do their homework. For this problem, we suggest giving the child a small notebook to write down each day before returning home from school, the work he did at school, and what was left unfinished in each subject that day. If homework is assigned, she should write them down while she is at school in the same book. It is your responsibility to record this information. At the end of the week, the parent should contact the child's teacher to ensure that the child has accurately recorded the work completed, the daily work he did not complete at school, and the assignments assigned.

CONCLUSION

As a close parent to children with ASD or ADHD, your role is extremely important, even if it doesn't show it. Your main purpose will be to explain or translate the complexities of the neurotypical world to him. In return, translate the eccentricities of the person with ASD or ADHD into the neurotypical world. You will be the whole world as a part, and you will play the most important role. Just as a foreigner in a foreign land needs to explain habits to a child, the complex individual will need explanations. Neurotypicals in our society need to learn from you about people with such complexities to be more welcoming and tolerant. Parents must do everything possible to help their children and as soon as possible. Some will be "recovered," and many will not. The goal should be to teach them how to make sense of the world and give them the tools to function in it to grow up to live independent and fulfilling lives. Helping your child learn by focusing on his or her area of strength or passion can make his life enjoyable and pave the way for him to connect with other people and possibly work in future years.

As a parent, you may know, but you won't always be in control. You must learn to recognize what you can change and what you cannot. And this advice applies whether you're thinking about a behavior your child has or a policy your school district adheres to. In some cases, the only thing you may be able to change is your attitude towards peaceful and positive parenting.

COPYRIGHT

This book:

POSITIVE PARENTING FOR AUTISM SPECTRUM DISORDER

How to Stop Yelling and Love More Children with Autism and ADHD! Peaceful Parent Strategies to Help Children with Special Needs to Overcome Challenges and Thrive

Written By

Jasper Hayward

This document aims to provide precise and reliable details on this subject and the problem under discussion.

The product is marketed on the assumption that no officially approved bookkeeping or publishing house provides other available funds.

Where a legal or qualified guide is required, a person must have the right to participate in the field.

A statement of principle, which is a subcommittee of the American Bar Association, a committee of publishers, and is approved. A copy, reproduction, or distribution of parts of this text, in electronic or written form, is not permitted.

The recording of this document is strictly prohibited. Any retention of this text is only with the written permission of the publisher and all liberties authorized.

The information provided here is correct and reliable, as any lack of attention or other means resulting from the misuse or use of